Gregory Gallivan
Health Care: Compassion In Action

Published by Spines Publishing Platform
ISBN: 979-8-90550-201-9

Spines

HEALTH CARE: COMPASSION IN ACTION

GREGORY GALLIVAN

CONTENTS

For Jayden and Danielle

Yea, though I walk through the valley of the shadow of death. I will fear no evil; for thou art with me.

The Lord is my Shepherd

CHAPTER 1

INTRODUCTION

WE ALL ARE ONE.

WE ALL need health.

We all hold health to be a self-evident, inalienable right for all lives.

We all want a better quality of life, love, liberty and happiness.

We live in a time of immense discord.

It is hard to find consistency without first establishing continuity.

To do so, we need to examine our common sickness that currently affects all and remedy it.

Regardless of politics, this is the time for isonomia, governance for all.

We all need a better future than we are living in today.

This is the health hearthstone of remedy for all.

In 3 steps, 24 hours to approve, and 2 years to implement, we all shall have a better tomorrow than today and make all the yesterdays matter forever and ever.

Step 1 – Use artificial intelligence for medical insurance billing and coding; doctors become independent contractors again. Artificial intelligence will streamline all patient care models individually, reduce fraud and waste, resulting in a massive reduction in health care costs and possible elimination or drastic decrease of medical underwriting divisions.

Step 2 – Education plan reform with a fourth-grade initiative to middle school beginners' classes to free college for all premed, nursing, veterinary and agrarian undergraduate students at all state colleges and universities; 1 percent given back for life by all students in the program to an independent body of a Clean the Universe Foundation; this highly inclusive plan leads to equality of opportunity for all students for the rest of time.

Step 3 – A round table of health, sincerely one for all and all for one; insurance companies crossing state lines without impeding federalism, permitting our implementation in states.

We need to find our faith again in ourselves and each other. For this, we need a strong foundation; a healthier structure for health itself provides the hearthstone necessary for this foundation to be poured. This starts with cleaning the stone, not replacing it, setting things up for the short-term and long-term views and eventually even a grand view. We will be artisans building and remodeling the hearthstone of health so that the stone is set properly and permits the foundation and all else built upon it to resonate properly for our individual and collective futures. This is the time to build and do what needs to be done. For each of us to find our path to independence, this is the time for us to move forward as one team united in our collective tomorrow.

Can one imagine the new ideas that can emanate from commencing this process?

Destiny awaits.

In two years, what artificial intelligence will be able to do is unfathomably difficult to understand. This is especially true in regard to just how game-changing artificial intelligence will be in the field of medicine, specifically in relation to how our medical and surgical experiences will be enhanced.

Picture a doctor leaving the operating room after a successful surgery; he or she throws his or her gloves up in the air, and this is what artificial intelligence will be able to do two years from now before those gloves hit the ground:

Artificial intelligence will be able to sense every move and action that occurred during the surgery, measuring, to the microgram or nano ounce, the exact amount of anything used or done during the surgery. This information can then be used to immediately document all procedures, tools used, time needed for use of the operating facilities, and all other billable occurrences.

The AI, fed with all previous knowledge of the patient from their medical records already being saved for cheap on the AI, will then be able to produce immediate, individualized, streamlined care that expedites the time to direct care received by each and every patient.

The AI will be able to immediately sense all the needs of the patient. Artificial intelligence will immediately schedule all follow-up care and any additional appointments, if applicable. All lab results and notes for care will be instantaneously sent to all necessary doctors, nurses, administrators and anyone else who must be informed, with AI knowing to keep complete confidentiality while maintaining all pertinent security protocols too.

Artificial intelligence will also have done all these things on a quadruple or quintuple check basis, ensuring the accuracy of all information.

The gloves hit the floor.

This simple but amazing feat frees doctors to rid themselves of being part of a group and become independent contractors again, bringing back the day and age when you knew your doctors well in advance of when you needed them.

Decades ago, substantial increases in malpractice premiums coincided with new billing and coding requirements that changed the landscape of medicine. The new billing and coding requirements made it prohibitive for doctors to stay in solo practice. The amount of time required to act as the administrator for all the billing and coding requirements did not leave enough time in the day to still properly practice medicine. Even if all the billing and coding requirements were completed in advance, the doctor still had to go through each one, as the final questions needed to be addressed by the administrator, the doctor. The cost of outsourcing billing and coding to third-party companies also increased immensely. This situation forced doctors to form groups and stop being individual practitioners.

Doctors may not even like the people in their group, or even how the other physicians do business, but those are the people who do what that doctor does near where that doctor lives. It is a forced relationship of necessity. This can lead to an unhealthy environment in the doctor's office itself, which can cause doctors to quickly lose their incentive to remain altruistic.

Due to this, we are living in the day and age when you go to your primary care doctor 2 times a year for 15 minutes at each visit over 365 days. If you are sick, then you are put in the care of a nurse practitioner who, despite being possibly the most intelligent and altruistic person on the planet, has never been educated in medicine at a medical school. Then, when you are so sick that your health is severely affected, you finally meet your specialist.

This is because medicine has become absolutely about money instead of the heart.

This program balances the two in a commonsense relationship of responsibility, quality, understanding and knowledge.

Medicine should always be practiced with the intent of a positive result being the only thing that counts.

Towards that end, an ounce of prevention will always be worth a pound of cure.

It is time to bring back the day and age of preventive health care.

The savings alone versus what will need to be paid out will be massive.

This is accomplished inherently in the concept of flooding every region with enough doctors, nurses and veterinarians so that all life can be prioritized in a preventive care model of health.

In the future, you will know all your doctors again, from your primary care to your specialists in aisle five of your supermarkets ten years before you need them.

AI will permit doctors to be doctors again. Doctors will only have to concern themselves with being the best doctors they can be. This begins with filling every region with doctors, nurses and health care workers promoting the concept of preventive health everywhere.

Hospitals will no longer have to employ groups and will reduce waste and fraud. Eliminating old computer apps currently used in most hospitals that do not communicate well with one another will save money and lead to faster care for the patient. Streamlined care for the patient will increase consumer confidence and give patients cost reductions. There will also be a reduction in pharmaceutical waste and fraud. Insurance companies will also save on waste and fraud and could have the possible removal of underwriting divisions or, at least, minimization of the cost of the department.

Patients will benefit from all aspects of this model and be given the opportunity to have the greatest gift, time, be on the patient's side by both receiving expedited care during the process and, ideally, having time ahead in life as the result.

By utilizing AI, patients will have customizable individual care models that fit them for the person they are. All aspects of care will be facilitated for every patient. Money will be saved by the patients, hospitals, insurance companies and pharmacies. Doctors will be permitted to earn their worth as individuals. The benefits will be reaped by all.

For this plan to work, we must have enough doctors and nurses to fill every area of the country. Education reform will bring true equality.

This fall, we will introduce a program that will start in two years for all fourth-grade students. These students will be given the opportunity to take part in a program in middle school, much like kids who currently take language classes, in which they will receive appropriate education that will culminate in their ability to attend college.

Regardless of any other circumstances, all children will be free to pursue their own further education in the fields of premed, nursing, veterinary and agrarian studies. This realizes our forefathers' dream of equality in action for all children for eternity. Once again, regardless of any circumstances, all children will be empowered, knowing that they are free to choose their own further education in these health-related fields. This realizes that dream of equality forever and ever.

The program will commence with age-appropriate courses such as anatomy and physiology while including courses that will lead to the ability to attend college for predetermined majors in premed, nursing, agrarian studies or veterinary school. The intent would be to create a vocational approach to health care education with a high likelihood of success. The only difference is that these educational environments will be foundational to postgraduate students.

The only debt that each student would be responsible for is their postgraduate studies. The likelihood of paying that student loan off would be high, as the undergraduate degree would be obtained prior to accepting that student loan debt.

University studies currently show that around 38% of the country has achieved a four-year college degree. The mark has been in the 30 plus percent range since 2011. Since then, of that population, just over 25% work in the field in which they majored.i That is a terrible return on investment that also leads to other financial concerns, including loan defaults and poor economic wellbeing for individuals and their families.

Vocational studies established early and leading to a degree would most likely result in a much higher percentage of students successfully completing university studies rather than qualifying to be on state aid insurance. There would also be a higher percentage of people who work in their field of study.

In this program, each child will have multiple opportunities for financial performance in various fields of pursuit in the field of health. If successful, the reduction in the number of people on state insurance will defray costs for all state educational programs from sixth grade through college. The tax revenue that would be created for each state should be a substantial quantity of proceeds. The quantity of revenue generated during each reporting period should be estimated to increase exponentially over the forecast period too.

Educational opportunities for children should never be restricted; all children will have educational formats available to them, no matter what language they speak or religion they practice. This will include Braille and other visual aid devices of learning for visually impaired students and hearing aid devices of learning for hearing impaired students. The pace of learning will be streamlined and individualized to enhance every growth potential opportunity possible for every student while never limiting a child's ability to progress at their own speed of learning. One such enhancement will be smaller classroom settings with fewer students per teacher in each classroom. This will require more teachers as many more students will be attending and able to participate with hope in their hearts. Also, since every student's learning style is different, this will provide different experiences and different environments for learning permissive of all learning styles and paces.

Quality education will become available in many places and at different time structures, permitting those who would otherwise be expected not to be able to take advantage of the educational programs to attend.

States and insurance companies will be able to realize the rule of large numbers being applied to their businesses. With all the health and safety advantages being put into place with this program, it is reasonable to assume that this program will lead to an increase in the need for other employees to meet the demands of quality improvement. This alone will result in a decrease in the number of people who are qualified to receive state aid and who are currently dependent on state institutions.

In addition, there will be several opportunities for all employees to qualify for quality improvement education opportunity programs in the health care industry. Working your way through from the beginning to the pinnacle of wealth management prospects will be possible for all employees in the health care industry.

In fact, all people alive currently will qualify for these opportunities. We will henceforth be known as the generation of health. Weekend and summer classes will be established to provide as many opportunities as possible for all students to avail themselves of in high school and will be open to all students. Official documents will be necessary.

Competition in the classroom will lead to meritocracy for participation in the fields of engineering, quantitative mechanics, zoology, artificial intelligence, aquaculture, and all other fields, too, rather than just the medical industry. Knowledge and literacy are qualities that enhance attitudes such as understanding and motivation. This boom in education will lead to massive amounts of opportunities and tax revenue while severely reducing the amount of unemployment.

Every student in the program will give 1% of gross income back each year for life, matched by a 1% tax deduction. This will be regardless of whatever field of endeavor is pursued after initiating enrollment into the program, including all non-medical fields as well. This fund will be a separate fund from all other funds from every country and entity in the world, including the United Nations. It will be totally independent. The United States will lead the way for all nations to join in together as one united cause for health for our planet Earth by donating this 1% tax collection to the Clean the Universe fund, with the rest of the world being free to join at any time. Those countries will have the same expectations. The money will go into an investment to earn interest as it is utilized as a clean world foundation. There will be a five-year moratorium period before the funds accumulated may be utilized.

A new management team is essential for a true bipartisan infrastructure to provide the urgent care needed to address multiple issues. Compliance specialists will be critical for analyzing the value of each action in relation to the allocation of funds for all portions of each part of the Clean the Universe fund. The goal will always be maximizing resources everywhere and doing so by always getting the most value for the dollar, or what is called bang for the buck. Independent and proud, the Clean the Universe Foundation will help to lead us on a journey to the infinite for eternity.

Every penny will be used to clean, provide therapy for and learn from our oceans, open land, deserts, highways, towns and cities. Agricultural farming land will also be included to promote clean food. Cleanliness itself is a foundation of health. Once again, rather than arguing the merits of cause, the answer here is again only remedy. Clean water, air and land will all help health.

Part of endeavoring to do so will always be studying the underlying causes of unhealthy living conditions so that preventive measures are in place if possible. Towards this end, large businesses will be able to establish new facilities that will provide a foundation for life in unincorporated and uninhabited areas of our oceans and deserts. We will be able to construct buildings that will be self-sufficient and sustainable independently. These facilities will be operated centrally at the local level. Resources for aid will be given free of charge from the Clean the Universe Foundation.

Before the end of the moratorium, these facilities will be ready for use. The idea of these facilities can be taken from conceptual design to fruition of creation, and the facilities may be operating at maximum capacity. This feat of engineering and building is important. It provides a valuable learning experience itself and will be providing prospects in terms of new opportunities for employment in new fields of study. Vocational study programs will be available for families at these facilities, as will all other universities' study programs.

For these centers to exist, an astounding number of diagnostics are needed to proceed with our quest. Each study center will require amazing achievements of knowledge, expertise, engineering, courage, forethought, perseverance, patience and ingenuity. This requires the establishment of new professionals, institutions and industrious individuals. New fields of exploration will emanate from these studies, as well as new career opportunities.

While the American flag shall wave first at each of these new centers of living and discovery as the leader of freedom, truth and hope for our collective future, let us welcome everyone with our arms outstretched as wide as possible permitting others to restart, lean on us when in need, and always feel the warmth of our embrace while feeling the beats of our heart now and through the rest of time.

Let us be God's helping hands and the helping hands that we all need for one another. We will be the synergy creators today for tomorrow, generating the positive energy needed for the complete repair of our minds, hearts, bodies and souls.

A new foundation of life where positive energy creation leads to threat reduction simultaneously, literally and figuratively. With artificial intelligence, we shall spring forth together to new ideas of harnessing volcanic methane gas vapor and lightning strikes for recycled energy use. We will find ways of using our ocean's momentum to create energy that can be resourced and utilized in other capabilities, as is already done in other capacities in other countries.

From the isles of Crete, Galapagos and Madagascar, from Greece, Italy and China to the continents of Australia, Africa and South America, we shall move forward together as one solitary team having one singular voice where the melody we create shall allow all of us to sing as one family in perfect harmony, or at least excellent if occasionally off key.

As we are all from this planet, Earth, we all shall be one in taking care of this planet. If the future holds the possibility of our existence on other planets, we shall do the same there. A refreshing taste of delicious victories together, emboldening our souls, permitting us all to be the child we are at heart and dream like we have not in years. Every one of us having our focus filled with a luminosity that brightens the path ahead.

This book is a new health care proposal that also reinvigorates the economy, creates employment opportunities, generates new fields for exploration, revitalizes the field of health care, restores health to the planet and creates equality for all permanently. This plan creates a true egalitarian society with real equal opportunity in action for all. If we up our drive individually, we will be sharing success nationally and internationally. It is important to remember that it is one thing to get the person you have affection for, it is another thing to be able to keep that person as a part of your life for the long term. It is one thing to open the doors of the playhouse, and it is another concept altogether to make sure the seats remain filled, so the curtain does not shut permanently afterwards on the stage. Persistence, perseverance, communication and consistency are all necessary components for a sustainable health care program to flourish, permit all societies to prosper, provide employment opportunities and to formulate a world that becomes one with a shared sense of peace, tranquility and love that leads us all into the future as we traverse the Universe.

CHAPTER 2

MEDICAL SETTINGS

Our health care system is sick. The health care system in the United States of America is not working, and due to how poorly the system operates, it sometimes helps to promote making people sicker. We need a healthy health care system immediately for a day and age of true health care for all of society. From procedural problems persisting due to not getting to see doctors in a timely manner to how aftercare is often treated to even the common level of care provided on a daily basis, the health care system itself is ill. Our health care system needs to be healthier for all of us to be healthy. That starts by putting the patient-doctor relationship first again and building a system based on care, not on financial greed. We should all be treated with respect as the individuals we are. We are not just a number, we are people, and when we need care, we need to feel that people care about us. The current health care system in the United States prevents proper positive patient care.

Providing the best care possible for all patients will always mean that the first step of paramount importance for any doctor performing an examination is to start by asking the patient how he or she feels. The second step is the physician palpating the patient while listening to the person being examined to determine any noticeable irregularities just in case the patient is not aware of an enlarged nodule or some other pertinent precursor. All possible information needs to be collected by the doctor before reaching a diagnosis. Professional health care administrators often skip these rudimentary and necessary base requirements for assessing a patient in today's health care settings. Ego does not replace acumen. Pretending to have knowledge of a matter and professing what care is necessary without actually performing a basic exam is malfeasance. This happens all too frequently in the modern health care setting due to time constraints. The goal is no longer providing care; now the goal is about making money. The more patients that are seen in a limited amount of time, the more money that will be made. Taking time with a patient is a necessity to provide care.

Redefining excellence in care with mercy being shown in a clear way in a grand view for all is a long overdue necessity of existence for all people, as we are all destined to be patients. In addition, access to accurate information and proper administration of elite care should be available for all and be readily available in a timely manner as well. Total customization is a necessity when it comes to individual health care, with all care being streamlined for every person. Resuscitation of a proper health care setting is not enough by itself; to move forward rather than expire, a remedy with new initiatives and old priorities is required. We are fortunate to have found this ford in relationship to time for the opportunity to fix things now.

In warfare, the countries or sides that have the better technology almost always prevail in the end. If you think about the concept of people fighting with bows and arrows versus people waging war with shotguns, versions of military grade machine guns, or even now with nuclear weapon capabilities, it becomes a readily apparent concept to comprehend. In medicine, the better the equipment, the better the likelihood of conquering the enemies known as disease, epidemics, cancer, plagues, famine and even for defeating death itself.

The safe caregiving needs that we are undertaking in our medical settings will require hard workers who are dedicated to continuing to strengthen the quality of nursing. It is important that nurses, doctors, administrators and all caregivers have knowledge that permits the highest quality of care possible to be provided in every circumstance. There is a need for a significant number of health care workers right now. The truth is that the more individuals we have in the industry, the more care that can be provided for all patients. Additionally, the more quality alternatives that are available and the more quality professionals that are accessible, the better the care will be for everyone permanently.

Strong communication is necessary for the successful implementation of robust care that delivers for our patients in the medical setting and for our children in all settings. The ability to convey thoughts, information and ideas about care so that the message intended by the patient or the doctor is also the message received by the other party, clearly and with the significance envisioned, is vital for success in all activities, especially health care. This should be what all levels of service in the health care industry are always trying to achieve in every correspondence. This means that there needs to be communication between patients and health care providers about what services are available and what costs are associated with those services, with each person's insurance coverage being assessed.

Solid communication is the ability to clearly, concisely, and accurately convey information, ideas and emotions while ensuring the receiver understands the intended message. This requires fostering engagement and active listening. Strong communication combines verbal, nonverbal, and written skills to create mutual understanding, build trust, and produce the desired response, which in this case is positivity for all people in the future. A healthy nation and a healthy world population inhabiting a healthy planet for the rest of time are worthwhile investments in making and maintaining the efforts that will be needed to succeed in the short term and that are also a priority for the ability to obtain long-term victory. The idea needs to be real in action, consistent with daily necessity for our triumph.

People need to have access to information on mainstream health care. This provides the first layer of data necessary to deliver services quickly and efficiently. Every patient is responsible for taking care of himself or herself and knowing where to find trustworthy info helps. Patients are in need of customized strategies for providing services that are streamlined specifically for the individual. Another common problem is overnight care, as patients are often exposed to conditions that are not up to date. Often, facilities have a room or two that are state-of-the-art, whereas the majority of the facility is not updated. In other instances, apparatus may be severely outdated. Information, good care settings and modernized health care equipment normally facilitate a patient's recovery and prognosis.

Coordination with colleagues is always an important part of providing the best care possible. The services necessary to provide the best possible care include quality insurance, education, training and professional development experience. Hands-on learning should be required under the direction of a professional practitioner, qualified representative or licensed knowledge specialist. For many people now, the options for care are being eliminated as some hospitals are forcing other regional hospitals out of business. In addition, these major hospitals that are left are now replacing their primary care doctors with nurse practitioners or physician assistants who have never received a formal medical school education. The coordination of care requires an understanding of the entirety of the human condition, including the body. Having an idea of how the left hand and the right hand both operate separately and together is a good idea. Eliminating primary care physicians from the field of medicine will inevitably lead to a diminished health care environment for all patients.

In all medical settings, there is a necessity for understanding the needs each individual patient has and providing the care each patient requires. Understaffing is a major problem. There needs to be more health care workers as fast as possible to be able to provide the services patients need. Right now, most health care staff workers are overwhelmed. What separates and sets apart most health care workers from the rest of the societal community is often their level of altruism. Simply put, it is hard to maintain a high degree of altruism when you are overwhelmed. This is exactly what leads to burnouts and high turnover in health care settings. Often, patients mistake the caregiver being overwhelmed for a lack of care, empathy or sympathy. A feeling of apathy begins for many health care professionals with a sense of not being valued or feeling as though there is no sense of appreciation, in addition to being understaffed, overworked and underpaid. A feeling of not being appreciated is something way too common in too many work environments now.

A community home care constitution is needed for patients and their families, as well as the staff. Home care workers are often overwhelmed with the amount of care they need to provide within their field as well. The number of people available who are employed nationally is significantly reduced from the number of people who are in need of assistance. The quality of the employment agency and the quality of each individual caregiver are also important. We need to raise our game for the elderly. The standard of care in most assisted living facilities has to improve dramatically.

While some people worry about the Amish and their health care proclivities, the reality is that there are pros and cons to the Amish system of health care when compared to mainstream society. The system being discussed moving forward has some similarities and differences in context and concepts. The Amish notion of health care begins with not over seeking care, especially when unnecessary, going with the least invasive methodology prior to accepting more extreme measures of surgical care, and starting care with medications that are the least invasive methodology possible until more potent medications are recommended. The diabetes rate for the Amish is only 2% versus the rest of society at 8%, heart attack rates are at 1% for the Amish versus 6% for mainstream society and high blood pressure is at 11% for the Amish versus 31% for most of the population. Amish people are likely to go to the hospital at a rate of only 25% versus the rest of the population.ii iii Their biggest secrets to the Amish maintaining their health are a nutritious diet and a lifestyle spent mostly outside performing difficult work-related tasks, mostly regarding farming, even to this day.

The problem with Amish health care comes from resisting care when care is needed. This is where life expectancy for the majority of the population has increased noticeably while it has not for the Amish population. Another reason the Amish population may have more difficulty as it gets older is also the concept of having a larger gene pool of selection. The idea that when people are exposed to more people as they go through life, they tend to build up more antibodies and immunities to be resistant to certain illnesses is true. This same idea is true with genes and heredity regarding having a larger pool of selection over time. A balanced approach of applying an active lifestyle and not over seeking care when young, while accepting health considerations earlier as we age, should lead to a prolonged life expectancy for all.

There have been incredible medical advancements in a multitude of fields over the past few decades. One aspect of medicine that is still concerning to most people is big pharma. There was a medication that was known to drastically help with weight loss and was marketed as safe for most people. This drug was considered to be a marvelous achievement that has helped many with their obesity, diabetic concerns and fat loss issues all over the planet. This medication is known as Fen-Phen. Unfortunately, when something appears to be too good to be true, it often is. Fen-Phen was found to cause heart valve damage and induce high rates of pulmonary hypertension. Some of these cases proved to be fatal.

Following a United States Food and Drug Administration recall in 1997, American Home Products, the company now known as Wyeth, paid billions of dollars to compensate nearly 600,000 plaintiffs. The pharma industry paid over $7.65 billion in settlements. The lawsuits were mostly aimed at the manufacturers of the combination of fenfluramine (Pondimin) and phentermine, as well as dexfenfluramine (Redux). This is one of the largest product liability settlements in the history of the United States of America.iv Some legal avenues for late onset injuries from long-term effects concerning delays in symptoms appearing may still remain open to this day.

What is the difference between Fen-Phen and Ozempic? While it appears to be the same craze, hopefully, this time, that terrible long-lasting unforeseen damage does not occur. Fen-Phen used stimulants to affect the brain's serotonin system and suppress a person's appetite. Ozempic mimics a hormone (GLP-1) to slow gastric emptying and reduce hunger. There is some reason to pause, though, with Ozempic, allegedly due to a lack of long-term understanding of what happens over time when a person takes this new weight loss drug for a long duration. This may also be affected by the methodology of application as well, whether it be oral, topical or by injection. Are these truly safe and viable products for the pharmaceutical marketplace?

What are the long-term effects of Ozempic? Apparently, many in the industry say Ozempic has not been studied for side effects that may occur over a fourty-year period of time. There is also concern that the medication could affect dopamine levels and the function of receptors in the human brain, which could result in a person's inability to process pleasure properly with normal function. These are valid concerns that require further investigation. The best way to prevent and remedy obesity has been, and always will be, a proper nutritional diet with constant exercise included as part of a person's daily procedures.

During the 1980s, doctors and hospitals started to get paid more than before by pharmaceutical companies to promote certain medications and were inundated with free samples of medications. Doctors and hospital administrators also received gifts, including trips, from the pharmaceutical industry. Sometimes these doctors and hospital administrative staff members, including high ranking board officials, got paid very well for endorsing certain products that proved to be detrimental to people's health. This was a large problem in concern to the opioid epidemic that was promoted by big pharma. In many ways, this exacerbated the problem and cost many people their lives.

Darvon used to be known as the little pink pill. It was described as a nonaddictive painkiller that was rather benign compared to supposedly more dangerous and addictive medications. This was allegedly true when compared with modern addictive pain medicines; however, when examining the reasoning behind the discontinuing of the production of Darvon, most medical research indicates this medication may have been far more addictive and powerful than stated while it was in the active marketplace. How do we know as consumers, though? Was the pharmaceutical marketplace telling doctors, hospitals and the average citizen the truth then or now?

There are certain people who have indicated that Darvon was inexpensive for a patient to obtain and was not as lucrative as medications that used oxycodone and other methodologies after Darvon was discontinued. This occurred immediately before the opioid epidemic, which has been proven to be due in large part to greed in the pharmaceutical industry. Many people are dependent on medications to survive as they age. Does a person really know what they are putting into their body? Does that person taking medication really understand all of the risks inherent in taking that medication? Is a prescription being replaced simply because it is less profitable than an alternative for the pharmaceutical industry? Once again, how does the average consumer know? People used to know and trust their doctors; do they now? Do you trust the pharmaceutical industry?

It is difficult to trust drugs being allowed and sold now when people who approved those medications worked for the FDA one day and then went on to take highly lucrative pharmaceutical company board member positions, often for life, afterwards. This is a revolving door that is much like the lobbyist system, where one day financial regulators for the government are investigating the situation of certain companies and then those same companies have the power to hire the people investigating the situation so that the matter is not pursued as actively. The same has been true with investigations into pharmaceuticals, as the person who was the point of contact for the government inquiry then gets a highly paid position in the company that was originally being investigated. The practice of people working for the Food and Drug Administration one day and then being bought off by pharmaceutical companies as board members for life afterwards is much like the revolving door that lobbyists in Washington, D.C., use all the time. This occurs when a person leaves a branch of the government and winds up working for the very companies they were investigating at one point, or vice versa as well; hence the phrase "the revolving door." This unethical behavior needs to end now.

Most drugs cost about $1 billion in research and development to create from start to finish for most pharmaceutical companies. Multiple layers of testing supposedly take place until about tier 3 is reached on each pharmaceutical company's own level of testing criteria before proper dosage testing is commenced by the pharma companies. What constitutes tier 3 for some companies may differ from what constitutes tier 3 for other companies. All this leads to the very reasonable question: Are these drugs safe for real? Also, even more importantly, why are pharmaceutical companies, the federal government and specifically the Food and Drug Administration inherently trusted, especially after releasing the opioid plague crisis on the world for decades in the past?

The opioid epidemic was a massive display of corruption and corporate greed that demonstrated that some companies literally do not care how many people are ruined physically, mentally, or spiritually, or even killed, as long as monetary gain can be achieved. Heroin is a cheap form of the synthetic opioid distributed by pharmaceutical companies, and it is estimated that heroin overdoses increased by over 500% during the height of the opioid crisis after some medications were introduced. Many athletes and scholars who had simple pain one day were addicted for life the next day and then had their days cut short because of an addiction to a prescribed medication. Hundreds of thousands of people have died because of this epidemic, if not actually multimillions, maybe more.v

The opioid epidemic was also the beginning of a massive change in the political landscape of how business is done. Most commercials on television now are from pharmaceutical companies. It is estimated that over 75% of revenue from certain cable television stations, including some news entertainment stations, is earned from advertising from pharmaceutical companies.vi

health care has become big business, and it has also become even more popular for criminals as a way of making money and laundering money that was gained illegally. Some doctors' offices and small medical clinics that operate in strip mall settings have become the preferred method for hiding illegal funds and having them returned as legitimate income. Even hospitals have become increasingly privately owned. The entire health care field has become a bastion of negativity, with its only concern seemingly being financial, not about providing care or health.

So many doctors and health care professionals, including an alarming number of female doctors and health care professionals, may be responsible for the genocide of a generation, given the many unnecessary deaths that have left us underpopulated for undertaking all the different opportunities that are now available to all human beings. Worse yet, the stigma and mental anguish that were created and never treated remain in abundance for so many, especially so many female patients.

This is in no way meant to ever blame the female patients who went through procedures at all in any way, shape, or form, nor the families or friends who gave advice. All hearts go out to them totally and without reservation. The blame lies solely with the health care professionals who did not explain the long-term psychological consequences and profited greatly from doing so, especially in a day and age where so many other alternatives exist. There are specific considerations for exceptions to this concept; however, they are limited in scope. Now, due to this program, all children will have the same opportunity to succeed, even including orphans or anyone put up for adoption. There also should be special tax break incentives for all families that are able to and do adopt as many children as possible. In fact, incentives for all families so they are able to adopt should be included in new tax legislation at both the federal and state levels, with every state deciding how much.

Some vaccinations are good; some are questionable; some are good for certain people and inappropriate for other people. Vaccinations are something that should be examined through individual necessities by everyone. Each person may have a different reaction to some vaccinations due to hereditary and other medical concerns of varying consequence. Covid vaccinations are constructed differently from measles vaccinations and were not tested as thoroughly before being administered. The measles vaccination is highly effective for children and should be taken, it would appear, in most instances. The Covid vaccination is possibly responsible for causing numerous cases of myocarditis in many young men. The rate at which vaccinations are applied may also play a role in the development of health complications, especially in our youth. Vaccinations would be a wonderful way to create a nanotech delivery system that could be utilized for each human body as a system for analysis and aid for care when necessitated.

Prior to Covid, life expectancy went down for the first time in human history.vii Why was that the case in a day and age when techniques, equipment and training had never been better before? One possible cause is that the Affordable Care Act itself regulated the insurance market into a money-making, for-profit industry that did not prioritize actual care for the patients. Many have referred to the Affordable Care Act as insurance for all and care for none. Some have recognized that the plans are better for the indignant through government insurance such as Medicaid in terms of covered procedures than they are for people buying individual plans in the insurance marketplace. Of course, it is hard for a dead patient to claim malpractice or complain that their insurance was inadequate. This is also especially true when someone is alive and becomes addicted to certain substances, as coverage can be exceptionally limited in such instances. Was there a direct correlation between the increase in various prescription medications and the decrease in life expectancy?

Allegedly, several medical professionals and institutions received a $500 Covid death bonus that was offered for every death that was listed as Covid.viii The expected rates of people succumbing to certain other illnesses and diseases dropped precipitously during this time. Did this really happen? If so, who was paying the extra $500? Were they the source of the disease? Were they the source of the vaccine? Was the directive purposeful so that more vaccinations could be sold to the government? What were the actual numbers of fatalities and illnesses that were actually linked to Covid? How badly did the entire Covid illness throw off morbidity and mortality rates? How long of a period of time were statistics not properly reported for illnesses? Why are there still currently bonuses being paid to some doctors for vaccine distribution? How necessary are these medications? How necessary are these vaccines? What other policies were enacted during Covid that are still being exploited? Why were churches closed, and strip clubs open during Covid? Was there a purposeful attack on decency and morality that has led to a lessened state of civility? What proof is there that there is even an issue with Covid currently? Is Covid still a potent health issue?

The morbidity and mortality rate statistics were thrown off during this time, as they did not accurately portray what people may have actually died from during that period. For instance, deaths from the common flu went way down during this time, and deaths from other diseases did as well.ix It is most likely that the incentive provided an opportunity for what resulted in misleading or even completely erroneous morbidity and mortality rate information to be accumulated during that time period. It makes what was already a declining age of life expectancy harder to establish in cause.

The reality is that sometimes there is corruption in care and compassion. The Covid-19 protocols may be an example of this unfortunate truth in today's health care field. Who set them? Were they completely arbitrary? The medical basis for most of the decisions made was complete nonsense that had little to no reality included in the creation of the procedures. While it was a good idea to separate initially, was this done on purpose to create a time when others who already had influence and power could reap unlimited benefits? There was a tremendous number of unnecessary medical gear sales generated by Covid. Certain industries thrived while others faltered. Who benefited from Covid and the shutdowns it created? Are those same people, corporations or governments still benefiting? Was this a purposeful socioeconomic attack? Where did Covid originate from? How did it happen? Was this a test run in advance of a larger biological issue in the future? When will conclusive answers to those important, basic, simple questions be available to all of us?

If a person goes back and looks at the texts from most towns that were sent out during that time, it is an interesting study. Examine a text or message received concerning New Year's Eve and the holidays during the height of infection. Most people in the United States of America received messages that said not to go out on New Year's. In addition, there were instructions that became arbitrary unwritten laws in certain geographic areas that enforced the maximum size of gatherings during the holidays. These false mandates were just the tip of the iceberg in relation to the forced home imprisonment of the entire country.

For safety, there were various laws temporarily put into place to restrict freedom and movement; however, how ethical, how successful and how necessary were those boundaries? It would appear that the states that did not enact severe separation mandates had infection rates no different from those that enacted laws about separating people.x Many people seemed to be bought off by making far more money from unemployment payments than they actually ever earned normally at any other point in their lives. Was this a purposeful act to stem any questions concerning corruption relating to Covid-19 programs? The amount of waste, fraud and abuse instituted during that time period seems to plague almost every state in the United States of America even now, with misrepresentation of programs and embezzlements, and the people in need never got the help that was designed specifically for them.

All of these forced instructions could be translated as an enforced law that states people should not have face to face conversations to discuss how corrupt this home confinement may be and the authoritarian state that was falsely propagated on the discombobulated society. A person's vaccination status should never determine his or her moral status or compass. Even worse, this happened right before a presidential election occurred that may have had peculiarities in the final election results. From paper ballots to a lack of people voting normally and even to possible ethics concerns in the voting tabulation, questions remain.

Regardless of political affiliation, such an instance raises the question: Was the voice heard from the American people genuine at that moment? It also raises the question: Is the voice heard from the American people genuine at any point in any election? How does one know? Nanotechnology could be used to reduce voter fraud, provide better health care and much more. The transponder system integrated into a biomass security system should keep all assets safe in the future and make providing integrity in all future elections simple.

The billing and coding companies that participated in the beginning of what reshaped health care into the current state it is in now were often originally owned by the same businesses that were invested in hospitals, insurance companies and the pharmaceutical industry. When a small number of people and companies control the health care industry, it is the people who suffer. A small minority of corporations deciding the fate of people by dictating how care can be performed by administrators and received by patients may lead to a terminal diagnosis for patients and the health care industry as a whole. The introduction of a single payer method would deal a fatal blow to the heart of health care.

Hospital monopolies are already ruining the health care industry. When there are no other options around for receiving care and a patient is unhappy with the manner in which care has been provided or with the associated cost, a feeling of overwhelming dread is appropriate. The business practices that lead to such circumstances in certain geographic locations in modern times are already highly questionable and are exceptionally concerning regarding the ethics being displayed by certain health care institutions. In some situations, it appears ethics may not even be on display, as concerning actions of selfish interest have been performed by some hospitals. This may be why some communities already do not have local options for their health care requirements. The idea that health care is about the number of people seen and money rather than being about the result for the patient can be seen in how certain marketing departments of hospitals function. While these sections of a hospital may not intend to have anything to do with their patient care model, the end byproduct may restrict where, how and when a patient receives good care.

There are rumors in certain circles in the know about how misleading online reviews may currently be versus the day and age of word-of-mouth advertising. Marketing is inherently a very different world in some respects from what it used to be. In some fields of enterprise, this has been exploited by some who have abandoned ethics, even if it serves to be detrimental to the community as a whole. Unfortunately, this now often includes the health care sector. There are hospitals that have used their marketing budgets in less than ethical manners of behavior. Some people have talked about being paid for a reference or a positive online review. After all, what is spending $1 million on advertising at $20 a pop for people to make up good reviews online, even when some have never even been a patient, when a $1 billion return on investment can be seen over the course of a decade, if not in only a few years? Eliminating all other hospitals in the region as competition can be a very lucrative investment. There also may be $20 reviews speaking ill about those other hospitals to ruin their reputations, and, once again, these may be from people who were never even patients. The idea of monopolies is not a good business practice in any financial setting; this is most definitely true in concern to the health care industry. Options in care providers are needed.

This is also, unfortunately, true with doctors nowadays too. Sometimes the worst doctors and the nastiest people are looked upon glowingly in their online reviews. In fact, some even win awards; however, these accolades may be bestowed for political purposes, in an attempt to influence which hospital becomes a monopoly in the area, or even just because of the person with whom someone golfs on a frequent basis. This is often done by some in the insurance industry and in the world of politics to force single payer health insurance as a concept.

Single payer means that there is an opportunity for those people in charge of insurance and medicine to have the power to decide whether or not you will receive care. Also, how good that care might be could possibly be based on whether they like you and what you stand for or not. Single payer in some foreign countries has even led to what some have described as periods of mass genocide for older people when implemented. This is a horrible idea that is often put forth by those people who are seeking to control people and eliminate individual freedom.

Single payer is usually propagated by the wolf in sheep's clothing pretending to be altruistic. In some instances, it is also thought of positively by those who do not fully understand the full scope of conceivable negative consequences and have very limited health care education. Fear tactics should not normally be used in discussions about what positive remedies there may be to fix the world of health care. While that is true, there is simply a sincere, unfortunate reality that if single payer were implemented in the field of health care that the fear that a person will not receive the appropriate health care when necessary is a real and valid concern. People should be confident in their ability to receive good care.

What started with certain doctors not cutting out all of the cancer decades ago due to the fact that it was more important to see large numbers of people to get paid than to do the surgery correctly and provide a good result for the patient has led to an even more egregious atmosphere in some health care provider settings, including hospitals. Being cash rich and morally bankrupt has been demonstrated as a way of life by some hospital chief executive officers, chief financial officers and too many boards of directors recently. Dead patients who received bad treatment have a very difficult time suing for malpractice.

The model in health care must become centered on the patient and the doctor again. This also means that there should be options available for finding the best doctor available. The hospitals owning the groups simply means that the doctor you are seeing is the one the hospital looks upon favorably as an employee, even if he or she is not the most qualified or the most capable in his or her field of medical profession. A specialist should be special, not someone who got the job because he or she was willing to work more hours for less money. We all need the best of the best to be able to become our doctors again. It is not just the field of education that needs to be revamped so that patient care is related once again to caring about the patient. The current model is money driven. We need to return to a result-based care format. We need to return to the simple notion of the patient-doctor relationship being the most important facet of what the health care field is based on for all people in the future.

The new health care concept proposed in this writing will re-instill passion and purpose in being a health care professional again throughout the entire industry. This positive environment will permit superior surgical care to be provided by people with big hearts and minds shining brightly and uplifting spirits. The world will be reimagined with localized medical centers with exceptional care and compassion provided by each facility. Because the details matter, this world will take time to create, however, that planet is easily imagined by all of us, for it is a simple truth of necessity. The reality is that good health care must be achieved, and, most importantly, it is sincerely available for all of us everywhere as of right now.

It is time for the individual to reign supreme again when it comes to providing care. We will all be patients at some point in our lives. Immediate access to quality care is a necessity for all human beings, as time is the most precious commodity available whenever there is a health crisis of any sort. This begins with reinstituting the simple model of what health care was based on when it was originally created: simply the patient and the caregiver, most specifically the doctor. The patient-doctor relationship should always be the basis of every health care situation. This modest structure is what the epicenter of health care should be, and all things pertinent to health care should be based on this humble model.

CHAPTER 3

TRIP TO THE DOCTOR'S OFFICE

For many people, the standard visit to a person's primary care doctor's office proves that the quality of the health care system in the United States of America has deteriorated substantially, especially over the past couple of decades. There is a fatal ironic twist reminiscent of the author O. Henry regarding health care as the current state of reality in modern health care is alarming. The health care environment itself has become increasingly ill. The search for health currently involves unexpected quality of life experiences that make an individual wonder if anyone in health care cares about health anymore.

For many people, this unfortunate reality begins even before they arrive at the doctor's office. Often, just going to the doctor requires taking time off from work and can prove to be a cumbersome experience. Important time sensitive work considerations may have to be put to the side. Other personal matters may need to wait or be rescheduled for another time. People may face additional peril while attempting to get to an appointment on time driving at speeds way too high just to cover the sometimes 40-to-60-minute trip to that person's primary care doctor's office. People do this because rescheduling an appointment may mean waiting for weeks, even months, for an opening for an appointment. In addition, that person may need care before an opening becomes available. Even if the doctor is worth it and he or she is absolutely the best and a truly great doctor and person, some patients literally have to risk their livelihood before they even arrive just to see the doctor to begin with. All of this is done by some patients to see if they are going to have good health and hopefully have a good chance of surviving for the foreseeable future because quality health care is not available closer in a nearby geographic location. This has to change now.

When patients finally get to the front desk of the office, there are frequently additional issues that arise before seeing the doctor. Understaffing of quality personnel throughout the health care spectrum has become far too common. Many times, people are employed with no previous medical background or training, let alone any experience in customer service or conflict resolution. A person may arrive to find that there may be no line and no one in the waiting room and be able to walk right up to the glass window of the enclosed area where the scheduling staff for the doctor is. Sometimes, though, instead of a smile, the receptionist may still refuse to acknowledge the person's existence for a couple of minutes. Once finally greeted with a curt tone of voice and extravagant, hostile body language, the patient must be patient and ignore such mannerisms to check in for the visit.

Then the receptionist may question the patient about routine things like the person's name and address three or four times, and for each question, the patient may calmly and pleasantly repeat themselves only to be met with attitude. The receptionist may then take another five minutes reviewing the patient's insurance information without saying anything. For many people who are elderly, infirm or injured, just standing at the window for this prolonged duration of time may be exceptionally difficult and even painful. Due to the wait, out of necessity, the patient may be forced to then put his or her things together and place some stuff down in the waiting room, as continuing to hold the items may prove to be intolerable. After being forced to wait unnecessarily, the patient may find that an ailment is really bothering him or her that day. Unfortunately, in far too many instances, this is now the norm in a health care setting. Intimidation or a power play is often presented first by staff instead of care.

When the patient returns to the glass encased area where the receptionist is, the receptionist still has the person's insurance card and driver's license. The receptionist may then get up and walk away to an adjacent glass encased room to make copies of the patient's information without ever asking the patient's permission. So why does this receptionist need to make a copy of the patient's most personal and sensitive information? Is it legal to do so, especially without any signature granting permission to do so?

Even worse, the information the administrator copied is up to date and is already accurate and available in her system. This fact was demonstrated by the successful surgery the patient had two months ago with this same hospital network. The patient's information is also accurate in another medical department of this same hospital for bloodwork. There is further corroboration of this fact, as the patient has a physical therapy department appointment tomorrow with this same hospital organization. If documenting his information again is done under the guise of a professional setting, that means that this part of the hospital for the patient's primary care has no idea what other care the patient is receiving through the same hospital. Maybe their internal systems do not communicate. His mother went to an appointment last week and sat there for over an hour to find out that she had already had the injection previously and that there was no need for the new appointment. This was a fact that she had stated to the staff when they called to schedule her.

The patient peeks into the other room and happens to see the receptionist put the copy of the patient's license and insurance information down but not in the patient's chart. This is when the patient notices that a doctor has appeared at the same glass encased window for the receptionist and is now standing adjacent to the patient. The doctor appears flustered and is asking where the information is that the doctor has repeatedly been calling this administrative office about. After all, the doctor states he has been asking to have the chart brought to his office to provide care for a patient currently in his office who has been waiting there for the information in the file for almost an hour. The doctor actually apologizes to the receptionist for having to ask again for the medical chart, as the patient is in dire need of care, which the doctor explains again is why he has shown up to pick the information up himself at this moment. The receptionist tells the doctor she has it and then hands it to him, telling him not to worry about having to ask for the information again. She states that this is because he was one of the "good ones," completely missing that the doctor had to show up in person because the information was never sent. The doctor takes a long pause, looks down, and then, with a tone in his voice indicating his patience has been tested to its limit, takes a very deep breath, sighs, and appears as if he wants to say something pointed; however, he thanks her and goes on his way with the information.

At this point, the patient is told he can "have a seat," and he collects his insurance card and driver's license back and does so, smiling while still in pain from his leg. The patient asks the receptionist at that time if the information had already been correct in the system due to the patient's physical therapy appointment tomorrow for his Achilles injury, to double check and make sure all is well just in case there is a situation where there is information that needs correction. The patient is told no; the system already has the right information. He is then told again in a terse voice that he could take a seat. He smiles, thanks her and does so. Although complying, he remains perplexed why his information had to be copied, why it is still not in a chart, why it seems to be randomly on a desk, and why his primary care doctor's office is seemingly unaware of the other care he is receiving in the same hospital network. The patient does not dare say a word, as he fears that he will lose his appointment. He wonders if the doctor would ever even know he was there initially if that happened. How long would it be before the appointment would even be rescheduled if that were to occur?

That was 45 minutes ago. The primary care doctor is providing care for each of her patients and is doing so without sacrificing time to make sure each patient receives the individual care they need. She is what makes this worthwhile. The patient does not mind this because he knows what level of care she gives as a wonderful doctor. The doctor's staff of her immediate care team in the office, including the nurses, is awesome as well.

When the patient is finally brought into a seeing room, he learns from his doctor's primary intake nurse that the people assisting around the team, though, in other words, the same receptionists who are the administrative staff, have apparently never let the doctor's support team know that the patient has called three times with the heart rate information that has been requested ever since the patient's last physical six months ago. Of course, this type of lack of follow through is nothing new, as a year ago, a training doctor was supposed to come in at the end of the physical with some information for the primary care doctor, and instead the assisting doctor just went home, apparently stating later that it was because it was the end of the day. This was a fact that the primary care doctor was so embarrassed and angered by that the doctor felt the need to inform the patient of what had occurred and apologized for it six months ago at the last checkup. The doctor also informed the patient that the person never took responsibility. Thank goodness the nurse doing the current intake knows that this happens and previously gave the patient her permission at the last appointment to call her personally on her cell phone to leave the information months ago. After all, if it had been bad news and the patient had not had that cell phone number, would the patient be alive and here now? This apparently "happens" a lot lately.

The questions asked of the patient that the hospital mandates are the perfunctory bureaucratic nonsense questions that cover liabilities for the hospital but are not questions of real merited concern for the patient. Even worse, none of the questions asked is the first question the patient was trained to ask in his own medical training. The trained patient thinks about the fact that patients are almost never asked the most fundamental question of all: How do you feel? Thank goodness his doctor will ask him that, though; she really is the last of the Mohicans. To this day, this should be the very first question asked by any health care professional in any health care setting and most people say they are not asked this basic, important question. Also, doctors should be palpating patients purposefully, regardless of how the patient answers, to check for any underlying possibilities of illness, defect or need of care. Left alone, he ruminates over the visit so far.

Ironically, the patient then hits his head on the hazardous waste box that is above his head where the only chair in the small seeing room is. No harm, no foul, though, as there is no blood, no hazardous waste needles fall on the patient, and the box does not break this time. The patient is not asked about hitting his head because no one knows it happened, since the intake person left a while ago.

Over an hour later, the patient still looks forward to seeing his doctor eventually to investigate what will be healthy for him as a person in life. The doctor the patient is waiting for is awesome, intelligent, caring, perceptive, and thorough. Once she arrives, the doctor will laugh and cry at these realities of the visit with the patient while both of their hearts break that neither the patient nor the doctor is an important part of health care anymore.

CHAPTER 4

MEDICAL ADVANCEMENTS

Joy for the best doctors, nurses, veterinarians and caregivers is found in delivering superior quality services that enhance the opportunities for a patient to have a positive result. A positive result is one that enhances the quality of time ahead in life for the patient while offering the patient an understanding and knowledge of how to provide consistent, individualized self-care. The gift of time is enhanced into something even better, the gift of quality time. Good leaders generally feel the same, as there are parallels in purpose and passion. This is a basic tenet for a person who cares about and provides for other people.

The advent of artificial intelligence will redevelop the medical landscape in a multitude of ways foreseen and some unforeseen. While some practical adaptations are already being incorporated into daily practices of medicine, there are still many exciting possibilities that have yet to materialize that will also help to define the future of medicine and health care. There are unlimited directions and methodologies that will be applied, and with time, even the seemingly impossible will become part of the ordinary for the entire medical field.

With the application of artificial intelligence, these advances in the medical field will take place in educational advancements, treatment possibilities, diagnostic capabilities, all surgeries and more. Artificial intelligence will inevitably enhance all of life's existence in some way, shape or form. There are very few areas of health care that will not be touched in some way by the impending realities that are on the near horizon.

New medical instruments, including new surgical instruments, methodologies and equipment, will provide opportunities for brand new surgical applications leading to other innovative new surgeries and new fields of study.

Glasses have already been developed to help those who are visually impaired and those who are impaired with diminished functional capacity. In addition, there are incredible new spectacles that permit the person wearing them to take amazingly clear and distinct videos. These may serve to provide a wonderful ability for many things in life, including for those who have cognitive disabilities. Prescriptions for these glasses are now far more exact, as they are streamlined for the individual.

Fiberoptic laser surgical instruments with an artificial intelligence precision guidance system for the least minimally invasive and most accurate surgical procedures possible will be part of all surgeries provided in the future. The new surgical equipment should provide better surgical results for all patients, in theory. The issues of aftercare with scarring will also diminish substantially. The ability to minimize surgical complications will improve.

New Da Vinci medical equipment may revolutionize the marketplace, as the company is already looking into ideas that may provide for a different level of existence than we have experienced previously to this point in time. The previous abilities to provide care to individual patients were enhanced dramatically by Da Vinci's previous marketplace creations, and the company's new endeavors may very well do the same.

Artificial hearts are already available, and in time, artificial kidneys and lungs will be possible as well. Developing better medical equipment working in conjunction with artificial intelligence will hopefully create a future in which, if there is a dire need, it can be remedied for good surgical candidates by changing out the old part for one that is new and works better, helping to reduce other complications.

Improvements in magnetic resonance imaging equipment are necessary and long overdue. Even the current MRI machines, open and otherwise, cause consternation for most who are subjected to needing care from such machines. It is possible and necessary to invent new apparatus that permits a more peaceful environment while still maintaining stability for the patient for a thorough examination. It may be possible to create and tackle new assembly utilizing artificial intelligence that permits multifunctional practice instead of using yesterday's ideas and being constrained by their limited abilities of technological application. Such methodology may promote a more comprehensive study into each patient's wellbeing while additionally enabling multiple studies to be conducted simultaneously. Moreover, improvements in magnetic resonance imaging machines in various designs would promote an increased ability to study and provide remedy for several purposes in the field of pressure calibration studies.

The remedies for renal failure need drastic technological improvement immediately. Kidney failure is a common cause of mortality and a very cruel way to go, as the body seems to just give up on the individual who suffers from such affliction. While the efficiency of the machines has improved since dialysis was invented in 1943 and was first successful in 1945, the method remains the same and is barbaric in its application. Many patients have difficulty in being strong enough to even continue the constant treatments. The survival rate for patients is only around 40 percent over a five-year span, while kidney transplant recipients have double the success, with around an 80 percent success rate over the same five-year span. Synthetic kidneys using silicon nanotechnology for blood filtration to purify the toxins out of a human being's bloodstream will provide increased life span longevity while also promoting better quality of existence with that extension of time. Transplant abilities are improving in a multitude of medical fields in relation to internal organ functions with increased availability. This method of treatment will be more commonplace soon.

It is expected that over the course of time, the development of artificially produced lungs will be viable for human transplant surgeries, providing increased capacity for life expectancy. These lung transplants may even be able to be done in certain settings of the body known as planes so as to be a more minimally invasive surgical procedure. Whether it be in Ludwig's plane, the thoracic plane, the sternnoxiphoid plane or the transpyloric plane,xi the ability not only to perform transplants but also to be able to do so in a way that preserves the original human organic material should provide for further opportunities for care as the individual ages and may need additional protection and processing through various new procedures that should be available at that time.

While this seems difficult now, as we look forward to an inclusive society where everyone is part of a system where health care has become a predominantly important part of society, this will become a commonplace, standard health care procedure that may eventually be dangerous because of an individual's ability to live independently and not necessarily need interactions with other members of the medical field to provide such care. Ethics regarding the ability to access and participate in such functions should be referred to only by trained medical professionals. Proper introduction and training should always be regarded as necessary. Medical training should always be undertaken regularly, kept up to date and continually reviewed for ethical standards in relation to the health and safety of all patients.

Artificial intelligence will enhance our ability to perform surgeries both in technique and with new equipment. In some places, people are already utilizing these techniques and new equipment to perform surgeries. New surgeries, methods of care, equipment such as X-ray machines, and new fields of study such as pressure studies and resonance approaches are part of the future. This will include vibration studies resulting from sound wave emissions, including possible degradation of resonance. Voice studies in resonance will help with all voice disorders that can arise later in life.

Artificial intelligence will also provide the ability to study different areas where stress is related to various conditions, such as internal stress and external stress. Eventually, there will be testing of stress effects caused by subcutaneous cysts, as well as of how cortisol relationships relate to synaptic function and how internal stress impacts organs.

Applications will include cognitive evaluation functions and aid people with developmental conditions and degenerative complications of cognitive recollection and physical movements. Diseases such as Alzheimer's disease and dementia may be improved dramatically with knowledge of referenceable cognitive function evaluations that were previously performed, with individual baseline testing being done from birth and continued throughout a lifetime. Research into Alzheimer's disease, as well as other diseases involving diminished cognitive function, will also be evaluated and enhanced by artificial intelligence.

The corona radiata may be a place to begin investigation into the methodology involving nanotechnology that will permit such groundbreaking health care. "The radiating crown of projection fibers which pass from the internal capsule to every part of the cerebral cortex."xii This process may make it possible to see what actually happens during the course of a person's lifetime in conjunction with the understanding of how an individual's brain processes information and relationships. We shall see if this works and how well, as it may be an altogether alternative methodology that bears fruit in mind mapping, evaluation and care in the long run as well.

Remember the doctor's gloves hitting the floor? The future of artificial intelligence will floor all of us repeatedly. The future of medicine will be preventive care. In that model, people will only need to wear a glove at home to take multiple medical readings. These readings will include heart rate, detection of asthma, blood pressure, O2 (oxygen) saturation rate, temperature, hereditary concentration, possible cancer screening, various illnesses and possible pregnancy indications. Every finger would have a possible difference in function, or maybe just the development of the device will permit us to read all functions simultaneously, no matter how many fingers are capable of being utilized. There are already devices that do a portion of these things and can be worn as aesthetic rings, and other strategies may soon include glasses as well as other possibilities such as wristwatches.

Almost everything will be possible down the road with further advancements in AI. Most people will have the ability to have peace of mind in relation to their health status while at home, and that is something everybody will be able to feel good about. Eventually, everyone will have the ability to test at home for certain health considerations without any commute. Artificial intelligence will also be capable of providing reminders to compensate for any sort of diminishing brain activity. At home AI devices already provide reminders of medication. In the future, how much assistance is needed will be able to be adjusted according to the patient's needs and abilities for performing activities of daily living.

A nanotech emergency alert system will provide automatic messaging instantaneously as a problem initiates before the individual recognizes it cognitively in some cases. For example, if a cardiac arrhythmia begins that may culminate in a widow maker heart attack, the system will recognize something is awry before the human being is even cognizant of an impending issue at all. Communication updates will be sent instantly to all of the patient's family members and professionals necessary to provide care for the given patient's needs at that time, including ambulatory and emergency medical response services such as emergency medical treatment services and the eventual emergency room, if appropriate for care.

The system will also help to alert direct care supervisors like primary care physicians while cutting down on the time necessary for corrective communication that may be prohibitive in providing necessary care. Essentially, this is the modern beeper system for doctors. This nanotech system will cut down the time for care by notifying doctors and all care staff instantly with pertinent, exact information instead of the health care professionals being informed later of a possible correction that is important to the situation, which, in many cases, will significantly increase the likelihood of patient reunification with their loved ones.

Articulating how nanotechnology will be useful in the future means understanding that nanotech is already used for the creation of materials, systems and devices with unique properties on a scale that permits atomic and molecular properties to change. This enables characteristics such as strength and conductivity to be enhanced while also promoting increased abilities for various biological activities. Nanotechnology is the manipulation of matter on the nanoscale, usually measuring about one to one hundred nanometers in size. Quantum effects are able to be utilized at this size to create phenomena not normally seen. A quantum is the smallest singular unit of measurement of a physical entity such as matter, energy or angular momentum that can be involved in an interaction within a given system.

Advancements in the field of nanotechnology will help artificial intelligence map the human body. This will provide totally different models than conventional methodologies for creating baseline information for each patient for every application possible, from physical health to congenital cognitive function testing to anything else in between. Stethoscopes are still the right tool when a doctor needs to auscultate to assess the heart, lungs or intestines during a physical exam. Palpating an affected area is still the right method for initial analysis for certain conditions of concern. Nanotechnology is the next tool of trade.

Whether it be a physical therapy application, construction or even surgery, having the right tools to assist in any given circumstance helps to mend, build sturdily and do so more efficiently in almost all professions in life. Health care therapy will be facilitated through the use of nanotechnology in the future. Imagine implanted internal nanotechnology was already in the body of a patient before the person attended physical therapy for a severe injury. When the application of rehabilitation care begins in the future, the artificial intelligence will correlate the information being provided by the internal nanotechnology within the human body cavity with the nanotechnology in the physical therapy instrumentation being used to provide care. This will facilitate, coordinate and maximize the efficiency of the time available while the instrumentation is being utilized. Artificial intelligence will be able to regulate the instrumentation so as to determine how cold or hot a treatment should be, how long the application should be applied and exactly what areas are of the most concern. The artificial intelligence will then be able to use the nanotech to provide pinpoint appropriate applications to the affected population while providing ample detailed feedback for the affected person, population, the caregiver and all administrators. In addition, AI will also play a role in aftercare models being established by using behavioral biometrics. This will include everything from studying someone's normal gait when walking to all other innate, unique physical mannerisms inherent to a patient. This will allow for dramatically improved results and any manipulation necessary to increase all capabilities while reducing the initial deficiency that led to the original injury. From autoclave needle sterilizers to artificial intelligence, technological advancements have always played a significant role in the health care field. Nanotech used with AI will be the future of all care.

Artificial intelligence may bring transformative capabilities to being a caring parent for all. Baby translation devices may become a possibility. Imagine the opportunities for parents to understand what their baby is asking for or what is ailing their child in a given moment. The power of being able to help your baby when they are crying and asking for help, and of knowing how and what to provide to help with what is really the issue at hand, is almost here. Baby talk will be seen as its own form of individual primitive language. This will revolutionize child rearing. Instead of only listening to noises through the night, parents will be able to hear what care needs to be provided. The educational opportunities for the baby may be unbelievably enhanced. Learning may take on entirely new pathways with speed.

Supercomputers with artificial intelligence capabilities will redefine the world of medicine. Inputting all data from all previously recorded cases of cancer will help to determine pathologies for all people and determine early detection risk models based on hereditary predispositions and any underlying possibilities of actions that could lead to exacerbation, complications and even the onset of cancer prior to the actual diagnosis of the disease. This will also promote the ability to individualize different forms of cancer, permitting the ability to distinguish between different possibilities of various forms of the disease and the likelihood of onset of each form that cancer may take. Individualizing the different forms of cancer into patterns leading to detection and remedies that may be found is long overdue and an absolute necessity that should provide better results.

Using the same methodology may also permit the ability to diagnose individual forms of other illnesses, as well as augment the study of the patterns of nature and nurture that lead to various forms of several diseases. Lupus, multiple sclerosis and Lou Gehrig's disease (the common name for ALS, which stands for amyotrophic lateral sclerosis) are all diseases for which there has been little to no progress for years. The ability to remedy each disease will benefit substantially from the usage of artificial intelligence to decipher any patterns that may be resultant from the nature of hereditary concern to the possibilities of creation or exacerbation from life activities. Given enough information, it is entirely possible that a few short-term remedies and even long-term cures will finally be found.

Life is more like chess than it is checkers. Strategic formulations done in advance provide success later and, if done with the right forethought and performed with the accurate actions, can lead to inevitable victory. New medical issues come up all the time for various reasons, including those that provide little advance warning, and often come from nature and certain environmental evolutions that we may not have prior knowledge about. New information concerning lone star tick bites resulting in Alpha-gal syndrome, an allergy to red meat, would be an area of study where accumulated patient data may be beneficial.

Many breakthroughs in medicine come from taking a second look at natural or biological phenomena that we already know exist but have not been fully investigated. Science often advances not by finding something completely new, but by applying new tools to old, overlooked observations. Science exploration using AI may help discoveries in concern to microbes in relation to the human immune system, hibernation physiology, healing mechanisms, cancer remission approaches, DNA applications, the repurposing of pharmaceuticals, exploration of side effects, and even understanding the placebo effect.

We shall traverse the Universe knowing that everywhere we go we shall be able to greet whatever learners we will meet peacefully and always be able to say, we come in Health. The new insights we shall have will lead to incredible new medical breakthroughs that will enable us to transcend and eclipse all prior medical applications known to us at this time. We will achieve an echelon never accompanied by distrust or dissatisfaction. The honey we will forge to find will bind us together with a sweet stickiness and be absolutely delicious.

Genome therapy is the forthcoming dawn of a new age in health care. It will begin with artificial intelligence using the thought teaching of observational analysis that was first created by Aristotle. This will lead to the generational ability to splice genes. Most of this will occur naturally with RNA (ribonucleic acid) and DNA (deoxyribonucleic acid). The study of multiple layers of polymers will help genome studies as well as help to create innovative solutions for a multidisciplinary approach that will assist researchers in developing various answers for diseases and all new applications of appropriate remediation. The studies will also help to develop entrepreneurial industries that will shape the future of medicine, research, possible applications of remediation and development strategies forever.

Currently, studies into the CRISPR (clustered regularly interspaced short palindromic repeats) enzyme are being conducted to provide possible therapeutic remedies for cancer, type one diabetes, genetic diseases and gut health. Additionally, there appears to be correlative data that would indicate there also may be applications of the CRISPR-Cas9 genome editing tool for targeting and destroying viral DNA from pathogens such as HIV (human immunodeficiency virus), hepatitis B and HPV (human papillomavirus). Scientists already using the CRISPR enzyme say it appears easy to use and is also highly accurate.

Genome therapy is the future of medicine. It will bring unbelievable amounts of remedy for a wide variety of ailments, illnesses and diseases. Using our ribonucleic acid, which is essential for protein synthesis and gene regulation, allows us to look at single stranded concepts of genome therapy. There are many forms of RNA, and they will all be helpful in creating a healthier environment for the application of medical treatments and, beforehand, medical prevention designed for the individual. This will include the pairing of this information with the specificity of the field of expertise so that each portion of RNA, as well as the whole of all RNA for the individual, is its own specialized profession. This will permit the construction of new remedies and prevention treatment models never before thought possible. Working in conjunction with similar fields of expertise in concern to deoxyribonucleic acid will permit specific molecules to be enhanced so as to strengthen immune systems against various viruses and to provide individual care for any genetic history.

Hopefully, in the future, artificial intelligence will evolve to a point where it can slow down the rate at which someone is dying when permanent solutions of remedy are not able to be found. It may be that finding those answers also just takes time. In the interim, if we cannot find a cure as of yet for such things as diabetes and renal failure, at a minimum, the ability to provide better results through hopefully entirely new findings pertaining to new methodologies of treatment and remedy will be available very soon.

Some may be interested in integrating with artificial intelligence for enhancing the efficiency of existence, eliminating side effects from medications, elongating life and especially, creating quality time over the course of life. Artificial intelligence will enhance medical education programs and medical experiences through exploration in the fields of biological study. This will help to provide direct links to integrated care readily available for both new and continuing diagnoses of various medical diseases and complications. Dexcom G7 is an example of using this type of forward thinking in developing its platform for diabetes care.

Labs for bloodwork should be done quarterly, as they provide incredible insight into health. They will serve to augment baseline studies in many ways, including helping to determine when an irregularity began when trying to trace back the etiology of a given illness. In certain cases, this may also prove fruitful for determining the epidemiology for patients.

Less invasive surgeries are always important; so are less invasive drug applications and methodologies of employment. Medicating should start with homeopathic remedies before proceeding to much more severe prescription medications. This should be a step-by-step methodology of deploying care based off of individual needs and capabilities of both nature and nurture. Additionally, drugs that are addictive should not be an immediate recourse for an addictive personality if there are other means of remedy that are also readily available. Individual practitioners of holistic medicine (IPHM) and other licensed professionals will become the first line of defense with medication by providing homeopathic remedies that may promote better long-term health than current pharma applications. Taking a medication for an issue, if that medication has side effects, can cause other concerning issues to develop as well. All medications, including homeopathic remedies, should be investigated for any possible side effects. All applications should be done under the supervision of a medical practitioner.

Delivery of prescription medication to the elderly has increased in popularity; however, there are still some significant issues that should be addressed immediately. Pill container models that are already divided according to the patient's weekly medication needs are purposely packaged to be difficult to open to reduce the threat of theft of controlled substances. The problem is that most elderly people then have an extremely difficult time opening the pill boxes due to how tightly the medications are packaged. When it comes to this concern, many elderly people have stated repeatedly that it seems like it takes forever to open the pill box. Spilling the contents of the pill box upon opening it has also been mentioned frequently. This can lead to a dangerous undertaking of double checking to see if each day's medications are poured correctly by the patient. Unfortunately, the patient may have cognitive impairments or may simply make a mistake in judgment, especially if the medication is dropped or misplaced. Physical impairments may also make it difficult to pick up medication in such a situation. On the other hand, trusted distribution starts with a guaranteed and trusted source of delivery of all medications.

Thermal regulation studies will help to provide accurate information that will promote healthier living conditions for many people who live in extreme conditions. Inhabiting other planets in the future may mean surviving in harsh conditions for more than 100 years to establish sustainable existence permanently. Some people operate at different temperatures naturally, and due to this, people can often feel different effects when placed in various weather conditions and will react differently based off of inherently different complex abilities to regulate conditions. When extreme heat and extreme cold are examined, it is cold that causes people to die more often than heat does; however, individual differences make for very diverse consequences.

Humidity plays a role in the health of vegetation and humanity. Proper humidity and ventilation are necessary for vegetation to grow to its optimal level. Too little humidity can result in the vegetation being dried out, while too much humidity can lead to mold growth. The studies into vegetation will help to create abilities for vegetative growth on Earth and for travel in space and eventually for the ability to inhabit other planets as well. Towards this point, artificial intelligence is already being utilized by the United States Department of Agriculture's Agricultural Research Service to use molecular breeding to produce, process and distribute safe food while increasing crop yields and providing improved disease resistance. This includes optimizing production, improving sanitation and reducing pathogens.xiii

Humans have different susceptibility to humidity as well. Severe dehydration can result from humidity levels just as much as from heat and physical exertion. The combination of such things can even be deadly if not appropriately addressed. This is especially true for larger people, as even professional football players and other athletes have died from this combination. Further studies into genetic predisposition, activities and other health matters such as the aging process will help to determine which parts of the population should be concerned with higher humidity levels and to investigate appropriate individual treatments.

Generational splicing of genes will also be part of our food abilities moving forward. Nutrition specific food programs based on DNA and actual activity accordance modeling will maximize health benefits and performance individually, as they will be tailored to the needs of every individual. This should hopefully provide some answers to nutritional protein food shortages for the indignant. We will be able to end world hunger for all forever. Artificial intelligence food source capabilities using agriculture are being created through the United States Department of Agriculture, which uses the artificial intelligence institute for next-generation food sources in direct correlation with farmers and ranchers.

Pigs are smart, and sometimes the problem with an animal is not that it is endangered; the problem is sometimes that certain animals are dangerous, plentiful, destructive and can even cause death. Catching wild boars would be exceptionally helpful in reducing threats to humans and other natural wildlife in certain geographic areas. In addition, the benefit of catching these animals may also help to create a surplus of bacon, ham and pork to create an entirely new chain of food supplies.

Predisposition to obstipation and other gastrointestinal issues may be able to be determined years in advance. Early detection may be achieved by investigating proper individual dietary necessities and may lead to possible suggestions for lifestyle coordination that would promote healthier lives than would otherwise be lived by certain individuals. Diverticulitis is a common ailment that may also be affected by the ability of an individual's digestive tract; additionally, there may be common threads relating to predisposition and common foods that are more likely to lead to and even exacerbate an underlying issue.

Sushi may have varying effects on different people's gastrointestinal tracts and may even be a large reason for the rate of stomach cancer found in Japan versus the rest of the world. The dangers of eating sushi, especially on a regular basis, need to be explored further. The rates of stomach cancer and major digestive issues in Japan far exceed those found in the rest of civilization. Regarding stomach cancer, Japan's rate, for a developed country, is alarming. This is also true of other Eastern Asian countries where eating raw fish is commonplace. The rate of stomach cancer in these countries is disproportionate to the rest of the developed world and has been for a very long time.

There are also higher rates of other gastrointestinal issues found in the same countries where raw fish is eaten.

Sunshine, good food, rest and a consistent schedule often promote a far healthier lifestyle in all realms of life. From physical activity to an individual's mental health being well adjusted in most environments, balanced moderation can promote a far healthier life and facilitate spiritual wellbeing. Cleanliness, both in self and environment, also helps to promote a healthy lifestyle as well as giving a good foundation for attempting to achieve anything in life. Do not overindulge, and do not underdo. Moderation promotes health. Balance is the key to life.

Paper towels are important to have in public buildings, and especially in public bathrooms, as they help to prevent the spread of disease. Many companies with public restrooms have started to remove the paper towels from their restrooms in favor of air blow dryers as a cost saving move. Unfortunately, this is a terrible move regarding people's health, as blow dryers send particles flying into the air, adversely affecting air quality, and much worse, the simple nature of drying your hands with items such as paper towels also helps to significantly contribute to removing whatever debris needs to be removed initially, too. In specific instances, changes can provide wonderful benefits; at other times, though, these adaptations may not provide positive consequences. The key is understanding when, why, how and when changes should be made that may yield the most positive results possible.

Some job functions may be utilized differently in the future. Nurse practitioners will work as extension of life caregivers for all needs of a patient's care, with the goal of hopefully extending the amount of time each patient has and, even more importantly, increasing the amount of quality time a patient has in comparison to the traditional care model currently utilized. Midwives are helpful to pregnant women, and during pregnancy, all help is good help. There should be more available training to become midwives, especially in rural locations for all aspects of the birthing process. The term care assistant will become far more prevalent, as these people will serve to augment all care.

Habla Espanol? Parlez-vous français? Sprechen Sie Deutsch? Nǐ huì shuō Zhōngwén ma? Kya aap Hindi mein bol sakte hain? Btehki arabi? Вы говорите по-русски? Ar tu kalbi lietuviskai? Czy mówisz po polsku? If you do, how fluent are you in a second, third or fourth language? Are you proficient to the point of being able to convey vital medical information? Patients benefit by being in health care settings where their primary language is understood. This is especially true in emergency situations where time may be short, and the ability to understand the problem quickly may prove to be the difference in a life being saved versus unfortunate avoidable negative permanent consequences. This can be hard to do even when you are speaking your natural language, as dialects and vocabularies differ.

Setting up facilities in each country with people who speak the native language fluently in that country will help to facilitate the creation of the hospital infrastructure necessary in most environments worldwide. This will also enhance care in situations where it is necessary for staff to speak simultaneously to provide the utmost care possible in the moment. The ability to understand one another fluently and communicate with each other will be a wonderful benefit to health care professionals in all settings. This is the type of addition in forethought of how to present the necessary foundation for health care professionals and entire health care systems to be able to prosper internationally all over the world permanently. Doctors, nurses, administrators and all health care professionals should be encouraged to participate in the care provided with the confidence of being on the same page.

The new educational format of this program leads to an increased availability of health care professionals. The program will lead to a record number of doctors, nurses and caregivers. There will be a real opportunity for better rotations for all hospital administration, nurses, admissions staff, as well as residents and fellow doctors who are all employed by a hospital in all possible geographic areas due to a tremendous number of professionals meeting such circumstances, criteria and credentialing being available in the immediate vicinity. Burnout will be less prevalent among health care professionals. In addition, refreshed and rejuvenated health care workers may be more attentive to detail and provide an enhanced level of care versus being constantly fatigued.

Due to experiments sometimes being run improperly, perchance being conducted in contaminated environments, and being affected by other unforeseen circumstances that perhaps corrupt results, there is something to be said for attempting again the same experiment that failed previously. In some instances, the hypothesis and means of investigation should even be tested multiple times using the same methodology to establish the veracity of the outcomes. There does come a time, though, when experiments become redundant. What is perplexing is that, oftentimes in the modern scientific community, there is no knowledge of whether the same experiment may have been attempted before or what the results and conclusions from those previous tests were. When scientific investigations do not go as planned or fail, the findings are often disregarded, and the end products of the initial study are completely dismissed as irrelevant. This leads to a wasted investment of time, money and resources in the future when something is being explored as if it is groundbreaking and new when, in fact, it is passé and has previously been proven conclusively. This often occurs and is a result of the fact that the end product of a learning expedition was never relayed in a proper manner to the masses. A book of failed experiments from all known past research investigations is necessary so as not to waste resources on redundant trials in the future. This is not just a financial concern. Resources necessary for investigation, such as stem cells and other biomedical products, may be in short supply, and proper conservation of the existing quantity of these products should be safeguarded. Instead of wasting medical cells, bodies, information and all else necessary to conduct all present and planned future studies in a redundant manner in relation to experiments that may have been done many times in the past already, a catalog of all medical and scientific experimental findings would provide a much better basis for future investigations in associated fields of inquiry. An easy-to-understand framework of research collection would provide viability and verification opportunities for a researcher to investigate before beginning an experiment.

We must adapt as necessary and do whatever it takes. Similar to the Grosvenor's advice to the first Norman king, William the Conqueror, in 1066, we need to always be dedicated to the hunt. Towards that premise, there are also various other curiosities of interest that should be explored for their merit. Some of these concepts have been debated for years, while others may bring newfound information and even possible cures through their exploration, making their study vital. Every path should be examined and exhausted to see where it may lead us later.

Women's knees tend to take on more significant damage than most men's knees when it comes to playing on hard surfaces over long periods of time and during athletic endeavors at higher levels of competition. This has been demonstrated in both basketball and tennis players throughout the years and is sometimes discussed as involving joints. Hyaluronic acid, otherwise known as hyaluronan, needs to be studied in men and women to see whether it provides regeneration not only as a topical agent but also as a possible internal reaction for the recovery and regeneration of joints and neural recognition capabilities. With the use of artificial intelligence becoming more commonplace, it may permit many people, even some who are currently listed as disabled, to find physical therapy pathways that lead to functional improvement. These advents in therapies may also permit certain people to be rejuvenated and rejoice in their newfound health abilities.

There is a common belief that excessive soy usage by men leads to less testosterone production. Additionally, another concern directly for men that differs from concerns for women is the usage of pink packets of saccharin, which has been shown to produce cancer in male lab rats. Conducting studies on male rats is far safer than subjecting male humans to trials on this issue; however, the subject bears more investigation and research before definitive conclusions can finally be reached.

Independent research conducted over many years with female rats seems to show a possible correlation between high metabolic rates and the development of tumors, specifically breast cancer tumors. Water absorption rates may also play a role. This needs to be studied further through more comprehensive research that demonstrates conclusive data. If there does indeed prove to be a direct correlation, it could also show that individuals who lack nutritious diets, have high metabolic rates, and are persistently dehydrated may experience cancer and develop tumors faster than the average female person. Clinical trials need to be conducted on female humans to possibly reduce breast cancer diagnoses.

The plausible effects of metabolism and water solubility possibly contributing to the onset of variant forms of cancer, especially breast cancer, need to be studied immediately. This is especially true for the percentage of the population that is at high risk. This needs to be done in relation to both males and females immediately to determine real risks. Determining the susceptibility of a patient may need to include inherent hereditary predisposition perils as well as personal choices that may impact health. These studies should be done in a conscientious manner that emphasizes quality of life, with a goal of enhancing long lasting life longevity. Other lifestyle choices and factors, such as preexisting conditions, nutrition and environmental factors, should also be taken into consideration.

Additionally, rather than a flagrant disregard for the possibilities or the creation of unnecessary hysteria over conceivable long-term concerns, the effects of dehydration caused by alcohol consumption possibly leading to variant forms of cancer, including specifically breast cancer complications, need to be examined thoroughly immediately. This is a disconcerting issue, as alcohol also plays a role in metabolic rates in individuals. Since everyone has a different predisposition due to hereditary concerns, has his or her own normal metabolic rate, has different nutritional needs and makes different life choices, determining what the probability of cancerous formation is and also how rapidly things may develop is difficult; however, it is still obtainable with new fields of study. Also, it is theoretically possible that how quickly a person's initial symptoms of cancer may occur could be estimated and perhaps dictated by how often and how much alcohol is consumed by that individual on a regular basis. The consumption of alcohol may exacerbate underlying conditions of predisposition for susceptibility to an individual and accelerate cancerous tumor formation, which could conceivably lead to an early onset of eventual metastasis. All pertinent factors should be examined in their entirety for possible relevance. Alcohol consumption results in high sugar rates, which could accelerate complications from diabetes as well as other digestive and intestinal concerns. Cardiac rates are also impacted negatively by heavy drinking of alcoholic beverages. Also, respiratory issues and complications often result from alcohol intake. It is plausible that breathing problems, breast cancer and other medical problems and concerns are all directly linked to the level of alcohol intake by an individual. The resulting comorbidity factors from normal imbibing of alcoholic beverages for all males and females may prove to be conclusively harmful. In addition, any intake of other drugs may also increase the likelihood of progressive cancerous conditions or the onset of other medical conditions.

A challenge can feel overwhelming in the moment, yet it may be what is necessary to light a fire in us to inspire us to initiate action, and that fire may burn so bright that, when we are faced with additional adversarial conditions, it forces us to find the courage to have to overcome all adversity. With those new talents forged from a flame, along with the attitude of refusing to ever give up, the iron of our resolve is sharpened, creating the ability for us to discover unbelievable amounts of talent, tenacity and resilience we never knew we were capable of before. With those augmentations of gifts and our newfound confidence, success is inevitable. Victory is assured, as it is no longer a question of if; it is only a matter of when. It is time to eradicate cancer from the world. A new comprehensive approach utilizing various information and new technologies gives us an opportunity to develop novel methodologies in the battle against cancer. Using techniques, mathematics and new developments in the world of technology may finally produce results for finding new remedies and treatments.

Presently, some cancer cell degradation studies that initially demonstrate promise are inconclusive at best. In detailed studies, there have been methods demonstrated that show that using a specific enzyme may help to slow down the degeneration of a cell from cancer for a certain duration of time. Regrettably, after a certain amount of time has elapsed, all of the normal degradation of the cell that would normally show after the time span does still occur. For example, the treatment may provide the ability to show no signs of any degeneration over a minute in the cell affected by cancer; however, when the minute mark is reached, all of the normal deterioration that ordinarily occurs in the cell during that minute presents itself in full. These studies are more indicative of a masking of what has transpired than an actual solution being found for the time being. What is achieved looks like something for a minute; however, since the same ill effects appear in totality after the minute, nothing of consequence has been achieved, as there is no elongation of health as the same effects appear either way at the same point in time. This type of frustration with research into cells containing cancer may eventually lead to jubilation if the inhibiting factors are vastly increased over a long interval. These studies may also lead to the minimization of the ability for cells containing cancer to spread. The hope remains that similar studies will potentially lead to the ability to mitigate the formation of all cancerous cells conceivably. Stem cell utilization in conjunction with research concerning all possible zygote formation applications appears to be a variant of procedure that could assist in the portion of the process to hopefully reduce effects, including the likelihood of cancerous tumors emerging. This additional level of investigation may provide an application that would be an advent for promoting health rather than just inhibiting decay and may be a necessary component for stemming the tide of cancerous growth formations. Also, this is where veterinary science may aid scientists studying human conditions as elephants rarely get cancer despite their massive size because they have twenty copies of a tumor-suppressor gene known as TP53, whereas humans have one. Some oncologists are already pursuing this possibility to see if it may aid with future research and application for therapy.

The next step in the battle against cancer may be introducing the addition of materials such as nanotechnology in the hopes of making mathematics matter to aid science for health. Imagine if nanotechnology were able to provide information directly to the patient and his or her doctors the very first day that a cell became precancerous or cancerous. This would help to prevent the exponential spread of the cancerous cells theoretically and possibly assist in mitigating the spread of the disease at all. The glove that will become available in the near future to monitor all existing day-to-day normal body functions of the individual will serve as a double check to make sure the system readings are valid. This confirmation will promote the ability of the doctor to know exactly when and where such calamity began and to be able to hopefully deal with any concern while it is still minor in scope to reduce consequences. Being able to provide treatment as the first precancerous cell appears will facilitate all care for the patient in the future by reducing the likelihood of invasive surgery while increasing the probability of a positive prognosis exponentially in both the short and long term.

Reminiscent of the famous picture by Leonardo da Vinci of the man inside of the circle and square simultaneously, known as The Vitruvian Man, figuring out how to apply mathematical function in conjunction with care for the human body has been a pursuit of humanity for a long time. The picture shows that the human body is ideal, as it is made up of perfectly proportional parts. Perfect symmetry is something that appeals to most people. Math is a part of our lives from appearance to function. In some ways, deciphering the exactitudes of the human body is like figuring out a math problem; even if you have all of the necessary information, getting it exactly right may not be totally feasible. It has been said that it is almost impossible to figure out the direct correlation between the area of a square and the area of a circle of similar size. This is a result of the variance in mathematical computations, as circles and squares are different in area due to pi being used in the determination of the ratio of a circle's circumference compared to its diameter for all circles. This is because pi is a never-ending number that literally extends into the infinite. Artificial intelligence is able to complete mathematical complexities that are almost impossible, if not impossible, for human beings to calculate, and AI does all math computations faster. It is theoretically possible that once a supercomputer with artificial intelligence is uploaded with all known cancer data to date from all patients who are suffering now and those currently in remission, after having their cells mapped by nanotechnology, as well as with all patient data from all past cancer patients who have already succumbed, in addition to all possible pertinent data concerning both hereditary concerns and lifestyle to satisfy both the nature and nurture possibilities of onset, a pattern much like a Fibonacci sequence that would demonstrate similar exponential patterns in relation to the cancerous cells spreading in an empirical fashion may be determined by the supercomputer. Is it conceivable that the application of game theory and perhaps chaos theory may also play a role in the formation and spread of all cancerous cells and that the information being brought together may demonstrate a pattern of behavior that might provide precursor signs that would indicate possible onset?

Chaos theory is commonly known by some people as the butterfly effect. The general view of the butterfly effect is that if a butterfly flaps its wings today, it could lead to a hurricane or a tornado later. This is an oversimplified view that should be viewed as a slight, if not grandiose, exaggeration. It is effective, though, in explaining the concept that the smallest change or action today may lead to fundamentally large repercussions and consequences afterwards. Simply put, what a situation starts with may play a large role in what transpires subsequently. When the initial condition is altered, there is a high probability that the final product may change as well. In some ways, the formula of the equation remains largely, if not exactly, the same; however, because the input was changed at the beginning of the application, the outcome will be different as well. This can be a powerful thought, as even a small alteration in the beginning may lead to massive variance in the ultimate outcome.

Chaos theory is essentially math based on studying small changes in initial conditions that can lead to completely different results than expected. In many instances, the application seems as if the results are random; however, on certain occasions, a pattern may emerge, demonstrating a true mathematical correlation of ideas of implementation and a causational final result. Chaos theory deals with fractals, intricate patterns that repeat themselves at different scales and can yield massive discrepancies in final results. Chaos theory, simply put, says what may appear to be random usually is not arbitrary. Chaos theory is already used for forecasting the weather, analyzing the stock market, monitoring population growth, examining complications with fluid turbulence, and studying the motion of the planets, as all planets exhibit chaotic behavior occasionally. In the case of applying chaos theory for early cancer detection, the sooner that a cell is noticed to have become pre-cancerous, the greater the probability of being able to have a successful treatment result.

Game theory is a branch of mathematics that analyzes strategic decision making, assuming that the participants make logical decisions to benefit themselves in the final end product. Since the participants do not control all aspects, how they react and take action after an outside influence occurs is also part of the process. In cancer, the person will not be able to dictate how the cancer attacks; however, preventive and proactive care models that are adhered to for the benefit of the patient will play a role in whether the final result is successful. There are concepts in game theory, including zero sum games and Nash equilibrium, that may not apply, as human beings are not always logical in their behavior or their choices. The idea that people are always doing the best and right thing for themselves is something that even the individual in question may not always see accurately. Even still, the base concept of game theory does provide some insight into the idea that if a person wants to prevent or overcome cancer, then certain logical provisions will apply to what actions should be taken.

Game theory is the concept that a game is defined by its players. In relation to cancer cell studies, each individual is different; hence, how cancer cells may form and how they may attack a human body will be different for each person due to hereditary concerns and lifestyle choices such as nutrition, hygiene and much more. The strategies involved in how to take care of each individual are based on these precursors and are also a large part of what dictates the final outcome. The applications of game theory include, but are not limited to, economics, politics and conflict resolution; it is already used in the field of biology for understanding evolutionary strategies and social behavior. Game theory applied to help in the determination of how cancer begins should provide a path to aid in how to mitigate potential concerns that lead to cancer as well as how to treat it for all individuals.

No person has full control concerning the actions of cancer formation. Cancer studies and applications of treatment have to be dealt with on a situational basis for recovery, and now the possibility of prevention will be applied in an individual fashion as well moving forward. Precision by health care professionals has always been a part of the health care landscape. Cutting edge methodologies and tools have continually advanced the ability to provide aid. Mathematics being employed with new technological advancements such as artificial intelligence, supercomputers and nanotechnology is the future of health care. The new, improved conditions of the health care landscape being discussed will produce more than just a longer life span for existence; the new health care setting will promote a longevity of life full of productivity and quality of life. This is more than merely returning to a time of preventive ideology; we will be introducing a day and age of preemptive health care for all.

The introduction of nanotechnology will help with all future health care studies and applications for treatment. The possibilities are endless, including possibly serving as augmentations for prosthetic limbs and maybe even assisting with the ability to regain function for those who are paraplegics, maybe even for quadriplegics too. There have been amazing advancements concerning critical circumstances with various conditions over the past few years. The integration of nanotechnology will also serve to help with all forms of monitoring and provide advance warning signals if a system is about to fail or falter at all.

Artificial disk replacements and other forms of artificial devices that aid prosthetics may be utilized more in the future in conjunction with nanotechnology. Back surgery, especially when a body part is removed, such as the removal of plates, heightens the tendency for pressure changes near the spine. The level of homeostatic pressure calibration being altered during the attempt to correct an impairment may sometimes cause aftereffects that minimize the productivity of a surgical application. This may be especially true with back surgeries where patients often complain about pain, ailments and lack of strength after what is otherwise a successful operation. It is possible that a change of pressure surrounding a spine may lead to various impacts on the entire central nervous system. This pressure difference may impact on all aspects of functionality for a person. An increase in pain is just as likely as a decrease in pain after far too many procedures. The introduction of nanotechnology will help to pinpoint any areas of concern, detect any deficiencies and assist in regulating care for specified regions and the entirety of the human body cavity.

Graphene is two hundred times stronger than steel, and it even has a greater tensile strength than diamonds. Graphene is most likely safe for use inside the human body as a protective coating for all delivery devices of nanotechnology to be introduced within the human physique. Nanotechnology should be able to be employed safely throughout the entirety of the human frame, with a tech enhanced shine protection finish permitting fluidity and ease of movement as it travels through the bloodstream and all necessary organs. This will permit a safe environment for the introduction of the nanotechnology through various styles of initial submission, including possibly as an addition to vaccines or other medical applications. Graphene is safe for human integration and will provide an excellent shield for the encapsulation for all forms of nanotechnology that will be injected into the human body. It is always necessary to think of things from a worst-case scenario in advance to be prepared for whatever adversity may follow. If the capsule for the nanotechnology were to break, it is plausible that it could lead to immediate disastrous consequences for a person. The graphene coating should provide an extra external layer that will prevent an issue from ensuing or progressing. An internal secondary layer for protection needs to be provided just in case as well. Additional testing for eventual possible decay needs to be done in advance.

It is not enough to just show up and try to play; we need to be game ready. When preparation meets opportunity, it tends to create good luck, fruition of positivity and generally bring success. Our medical preparation needs to be first rate, not a last second thought, resort or a misguided reactionary response. Taking the time to get things done right and done so in an expeditious manner requires constant investigation and reevaluation to ensure substantiation that the process is ready and correct. Exploring each and every seemingly innocuous detail of the process may prove to be excruciatingly difficult; however, the reward may create a euphoric sense that is so invigorating it gets our endorphins pumping with an excited anticipation of what may be next. Upon reflection, the courageous pursuit of preemptive health care may one day be looked back upon with a high degree of adulation. We need to explore all concepts and see where the truth leads us.

When people say, "I don't care," what they usually really mean is they care so much it hurts. Usually, this is a self-defense mechanism that indicates that they care tremendously and are afraid of getting hurt. It is time to be honest and say that caring is a good and healthy thing to endeavor for in life. Health is wealth, for what good is wealth without good health? It is important to remember that, in life, the glass is always full, and to proceed accordingly, even on days when we thirst for more out of life and our desires cannot be quenched. Happy, healthy, cool, calm, and collected, we shall have the determination to match our strength and our intelligence. The colors of blood are the colors of the American flag: red is oxygenated blood, blue is blood lacking oxygen and lymphatic white defends our health. We all should be willing to stand up for our health. While our blood types may differ, it is how our blood works that shows we are all the same.

We all need clean water, clean air and clean land. From the poorest of us to the most influential, we all need health. Simply put, it is time to care about care. We can all use new, fresh service with integrity being readily available in our health care system, a gentle cleansing to refurbish health care into being about health and care again, where that simple concept is of paramount importance for the entire medical industry and for all human beings forever.

In regard to making the doctor–patient relationship the basis of health care again, we will do our best to return to the simplicity of the snake and stick, known as the Rod of Asclepius. It is the only symbol that is truly indicative of a surgeon. Its elegant ease is a wonderful model to emulate again.

Health care professionals will also be resuscitating the true original purpose of the Hippocratic Oath. We must restore the concept of benefiting patients according to the greatest abilities and judgments available irrespective of all other potential factors. At its inception, the Hippocratic Oath was translated very differently than it is currently instituted. The real Oath is about more than just doing no harm; in truth, the actual concept is based on doing everything a person can possibly do at all times for a fellow member of humankind. The difference between the original concept and how it is presently interpreted is as vast as the difference between night and day. When a health care professional demonstrates that damage was not done during a procedure, the actions taken may be very different than doing all and everything conceivable to help the patient. With the implementation of this new health care model, here and now, the original purpose of the Hippocratic Oath will be reestablished once and for all. Health care is about taking responsibility for another person, animal or any living thing and doing everything one can.

Saying we will help is not enough. Now is the time to take action in a noble venture for a legacy for all aspects of life that institutes reform of health care so that anything-anywhere-anytime available services will always deliver superior quality care for all of us swiftly with conviction as strong as steel. This should be done with a core covenant certifying our commitment. This is not just on an interstate basis; however, it is a true worldwide endeavor for magic to be shared internationally. We will be engineering, maintaining and finding cures for hunger and all remaining remedies necessary for all. We will harness enthusiasm and understanding and use both as we take that negative potential energy and channel it into a positive force with a prime directive deep in our souls, hearts and minds so that we provide the harvest we all need for eternity.

Smarter living is transforming the infrastructure of health into the infinite. May we never stop becoming more advanced with our health. We are all ready to be refreshed with good news. We shall create caring solutions for all individuals, including infants, children, women and men too, a power stroke that matters to all. We shall learn how to create and build quality beyond our ability to comprehend, like a Stradivarius violin.

There is the do it factor in life; however, equally important is also the to it factor in life. Success is dependent on both things being done and being done correctly. The to it and the do it factors both count. For advancing health care the time to get to it and do it is right now.

CHAPTER 5

MENTAL HEALTH

We all need space for growth. As discussed throughout this document, health comes in many forms. Questions regarding counseling and psychological services for mental health also must be addressed. It is important to stop being so judgmental, as it is often a sign of being afraid and usually means one is anxious about being judged by outside sources and influences. It is time to pump the brakes instead and have unlimited opportunities available afterwards. Towards this end, it is time to put a permanent stop to any type of mental health stigma. Seeking meaningful health of any sort should be apposite, and seeking mental health should always be appropriate and acceptable. When a person does so, this endeavor in self-care should be applauded and expanded upon in all reasonable respects for responsible prevention.

Generally, for those who are ill, it is difficult to maintain psychological quality, regardless of whether knowledge has been developed prior to a diagnosis. Rather than continuing treatment that proves ineffective, alternative patient care should be available. Typically, patients qualify for treatment quickly enough to justify treatment rather than having no opportunity to find quality care provided. The problem with care comes with the fact that most mental health facilities and treatment centers have always been understaffed, underpaid and underappreciated. There also need to be more mental health facilities.

Mental health for individuals can start to become a priority with less stigma attached to any condition, with 24-hour coffee and tea available at safe havens, including town halls, granges, libraries, places of worship and other spaces across the country where people can share ideas, concerns and feelings. No leader will be necessary, just a place for people to show up and share their thoughts as they wish with others with whom they probably have a lot in common. Cleanup and care with respect for the environment, views and each other are required for participation. These should not be used as places of habitation. These will be open, affirmative, all are welcome, safe spots that are dedicated to preventing mental health problems by permitting a peaceful environment for those in need of refuge. A place simply not to be or feel alone or forgotten. This should be one of the main functions performed at auxiliary Safe Haven centers differentiated from Safe Haven centers where children's and other adult recreational activities occur. The goal is to develop an atmosphere where community and wellbeing are enhanced by neighborhood participation in social interaction and integration. A licensed therapist should always be available 24 hours a day to assist with any severe trauma cases or any other necessary treatment for those medical conditions that prove to be more challenging and require frequent and further investigation.

Common sense is a sense that is no longer so common. While some people may say that common sense is no longer as necessary because artificial intelligence will mask enormous amounts of deficiencies and unacceptable behavior, common sense will always be a virtue of importance.

Knowing how to do basic stuff without overcomplicating things unnecessarily is essential for survival and for the ability to thrive too. However, the truth is that we all are prone to being the person who may become lost in our own emotions at any time. In any given moment, we all may not be capable of displaying or performing actions at that instant with any application of what constitutes common sense.

Lucid thinking is critically important for rational interpretation and reasoning for proper processing of both internal and external factors of influence. For example, a balanced resonance of internal harmony is only accomplished when proper interpretation of the surrounding environment and other external factors permit a balance between the action occurring and the variables of contributing influence so that success in having internal acceptance, logical reasoning and a peaceful mindset may be achieved. Correct reasoning is a necessity to attain a proper understanding of what our own opinions are and to evaluate our own experiences, expectations and existence to find our own optimal frequency of resonance for life. This is especially important because it is easy for any of us to lose our bearings as to where we need to go and where we want to go while we must go and need to keep going too. Proper internal resonance is a necessary component of mental health and a well-balanced existence.

Being consistent is harder than people think. This can be a good thing too though, as it keeps us humble. We are all human, and we are all capable of having a bad day; sometimes this is beyond our control. This is true from a day-to-day perspective and also may be relevant from moment to moment too. Event management within the individual can include having to be able to process an extreme number of different emotions within a variety of diverse parts of the environment that are dependent on various external factors that may influence the moment and our daily lives. This can even translate into momentary processes, such as stress, that can influence our individual immune systems.

Obviously, stress can cause a person to make better decisions or worse decisions, depending on other factors, including the nature of the person's situation, their ability to make choices, preparation, experience, critical reasoning skills, ability to process information within types of situations, background, and other factors such as the individual's living environment. Either way, it is possible to decipher that any situation can have a large effect on thought processes. All of these factors occur on a subconscious level before we even start to think about consistency of action on a conscious level because of these internal factors that being consistent necessitates.

Sex, alcohol and drug usage all play a significant role in the proper function of cognitive abilities for each individual. Substance abuse programs will start with local urgent care centers for alcoholism and drug addiction. The actual start will hopefully occur by reducing the number of people who become addicted by increasing the positivity and quality of time for all life. It is important that we provide relief for the overwhelmed. In concern to the fact that substance abuse can happen to any of us, we need to act not out of a war on drugs, but instead we must take positive action because of care in our hearts, as there, but for the grace of God, go we. Towards this end, drug treatment and testing will be available at all urgent care treatment facilities.

Companies may wish to employ their own mental health professionals to defray costs associated with care. Their employees may have a higher return on efficient time spent on work if they feel the company they represent cares about them as individuals. This can be accomplished by looking at ideas like giving all employees two paid days a year to meet with a therapist who provides care for the company regarding mental health responsibilities. Also, discounts for gyms and access to nutritional information demonstrate care for an employee. An investment by companies in the health of their employees, always and at all levels of employment, will be paid back in massive dividends of productivity.

Serenity is the state of being tranquil, calm and peaceful. It requires being committed to staying connected to your surroundings and environment, as well as being in tune with what can and cannot be done with those things that bear consequences. Sometimes, it is not that easy to discern, nor so readily available for knowledge, that consequences will even occur. It is helpful to have parents, or at least one parent, who can instill such a feeling of comfort and confidence so that the difficulties of life may be met with an acceptance born from serenity. Even then, the meaning of serenity is truly assigned by the individual and will vary greatly from one person to another.

Serenity is important and sometimes is simply known by some people through what is commonly referred to as the Serenity Prayer. In essence, this is a plea for God, or a higher power or energy source for others, to bless us with the ability to recognize what we can change, what we cannot, and the wisdom to know the difference. Our relationships with spirituality and our understanding of serenity are as individual as our fingerprints or our taste buds. A person must pray their way through life in their own way, whatever that does or does not mean to that person. Even if the person's methodology of prayer is to not pray or even refuse to participate in prayer, they are forging a path of their own for personal inner peace and acceptance. Having discipline is important to find peace, have a sense of belonging, and feel blessed.

Taking responsibility for our own actions and decisions is very important and a necessary part of health and wellbeing. Taking responsibility for our own actions is a vital part of honesty. Honesty is a major part of integrity. Integrity is a vital part of truth. Truth is important because it is a major part of health because the truth is what sets us free. This is true with our own selves and in any other relationship of importance.

Engaging in positive activities and making positive choices consistently help to create an environment of peace, positivity and health in each of our lives. We need to be kind, gentle and understanding with ourselves in a very difficult world to do so in. Peace and positivity will not be found by looking to the outside world to heal you; one must heal oneself internally to be able to function. The simple truth is that life is hard for all of us. The more honest and caring we are with ourselves, the better equipped we will be to be able to move forward as individuals and as a collective community.

Music and humor are excellent starting points for communication and health. The best jokes are the funniest because they have the most truth in them. It is important to learn to laugh at ourselves with confidence and with no ostensible loss of self-respect or self-worth. People should prioritize focusing on healthy activities that occur outside in fresh air. Read before bed to enhance quality sleep patterns. All of this creates permeability throughout the day that enhances the ability to go with the flow as the day unfolds.

It is empowering to be employed. If someone gives you five dollars versus requiring you to work for an hour for five dollars, in which case are you more likely to spend the money frivolously, and in which case are you more likely to put the money into a savings account? Responsibility at a young age, within reason as well, helps a human to develop. There should be a balance between responsibility, education, physical development, and psychological enhancement matched with the necessary quality time for each person to experience life on their own terms while also having as much fun and positivity as possible.

The truth is that there are many mentally unhealthy people who thrive in the real world. While that is true, for personal growth and long-term acceptance of oneself, self-regulating against dishonesty is exceptionally important in everyday life to be able to grow and function positively and properly. A person may not see the truth clearly; however, attempting to do so does allow for a healthy internal environment. Permitting a seed of dishonesty may allow it to manifest itself into a field of disillusionment, denial, dissatisfaction, disassociation, delusion, destruction, and possibly death. Some people are so narcissistic that they truly believe that this might be the end of all days because they believe that this must be the most important time in all of history because they are alive today. Narcissistic egos and self-importance have drained society through a lack of empathy and destroyed morality.

Rose, bud and thorn is a way for some people to figure out their day in terms of the positive, the negative and the ideas that give them hope for inspiration for the future. This is one example of practicing acceptance and trying to utilize the reality of any given day as the seeds necessary for the flowers of our own lives to bloom and be cultivated tomorrow.

Communication with others, when done with vulnerability and total honesty, can lead to the most rewarding, fulfilling and trusting relationships we establish with others in our community. Doing this consistently may also help to lead to reductions in the amount of mental health stigmas.

You have to move forward in life to something. You can never run from something because you will always take the baggage with you wherever you go. Gentle kindness, beginning with honesty with ourselves and appreciation for our own existence, takes each of us much further in the journey of life. Even then, it will take time and patience to see the total fruition of our labors. For even if success is readily apparent much faster than anticipated or expected, it can take a while for people to get adjusted to new surroundings and concepts. Even under the best of conditions, it can take weeks for the human mind to accomplish having its individual circadian rhythms adjust to any new environment or circumstance. It may even take a long time thereafter for the human body to be able to adjust to new conditions and environments.

People should be able to have the proper time to grieve without facing additional repercussions. Unfriendly as it may be, though, this is not always a realistic sentiment when it comes to the workplace environment. On the other hand, it would be difficult and maybe disastrous to return to the workplace environment too soon and not be able to handle the responsibilities of the job correctly and make an unforgettable and unfortunate mistake. It is important to have patience when it comes to getting over a significant loss. It takes time for the grieving person to be able to fully understand and accept the changes that have taken place. Even then, the truth is, with some losses, it does not get better, it just becomes different, and the difficulties must still be dealt with, accepted and addressed.

Personal space is a necessary part of mental health for all individuals. Personal space is the hearthstone of mental health. Simply put, when adversity inevitably finds us again, the most important and the best thing for all of us to do to start is to just breathe. Free air is a good thing. Personal space is necessary in all things, even in our relationships with our own family members. The group dynamics of family should never be used as a weapon.

This should also be applied with a reintroduction of mental health facilities that used to be much more readily available than facilities are today. There is a major difference in approach that should occur, though, in that these facilities should be created on large estates and in extremely rural areas. These mental health facilities should not be reminiscent of current prison structures, as they often are today. They should be in wide open areas where people have the ability to feel free to breathe and are far less likely to feel claustrophobic. With the ability of modern video surveillance and the future of artificial intelligence permitting instantaneous geopositioning services on any single human being by using nanotechnology, there is no reason to not permit such a structure.

In fact, most state juvenile detention centers should immediately take on this idea, and it should lead to far less recidivism for the children as they turn into adults. States could send their youth detainees to other states that have more space, such as farmland in Maine, Montana, Iowa, Wyoming, Idaho, Wisconsin, North Dakota, South Dakota and upstate New York, for a positive environment. Structure and vocational education should be available for all youths, so the idea of having people grow up to be less likely to be habitual offenders will be true. The investment in such a cost should save lives and money in the future for all of society as well. This will need to be balanced with a family's desire to visit.

Healthy environmental conditions should exist for anyone who is incarcerated as well. Prisons need healthy housing facilities that are better and safer, with more free room for all incarcerated people to roam when permitted, both inside and outside, when and where appropriate. There should be access to affordable health care for all people who are incarcerated as well. There should be a healthier environment for all involved, including the staff as well as the inmates. Tight quarters and understaffing can cause the prison staff to feel overwhelmed, which can be perceived as a lack of empathy between staff and individuals incapacitated from freedom, while increasing tensions that could lead to a catastrophic situation. After many years of working in a facility, prison guards may feel the wear of being behind bars themselves. More staff being employed, with larger cohabitation areas inside and outside the prisons, maintained by the perimeter of the structure itself, will lead to far healthier environments being sustained adjacent to the prison structures and within the confines of the actual prison buildings themselves.

We are meant to be social animals, and so, while free air and personal space are needed to survive, we truly need the rest of the herd to feel our best, be our healthiest, and thrive. There should be multitudes of mental health awareness charity baseball and softball games, as well as events in other sports too, held at beautiful locations. These charitable actions will work best if sponsored by both former athletic directors and volunteers, including retired athletes and other celebrities who wish to give back. This will be an opportunity to share stories of inspiration to help raise awareness and reduce stigmas caused by neurological conditions and other mental health situations. In this vein, an activity awareness day for mental health will support taking people away from preconceived notions and provide the financial means to support mental health programs.

It is important for us to foster and engage the relationship between parents and children. Positive mental health can only truly be found by finding peace with the other people who are important in a person's life. If the other person were to pass on, and you have not found peace with them, it is not the deceased person who is left to try and navigate their way back to a state of acceptance. It is the person who remains who must find a way towards love, tolerance, acceptance and being at peace.

Allow our examination into mental health to be as deep as possible, like the investigation we will be doing in the oceans, and extend as far as we will go in our exploration of space. Life goes by too fast to even remember all the things that occurred and were a part of our own lives, let alone trying to keep up with everyone else entirely. It is hard enough to keep in touch with ourselves with the limited time remaining in each day. We show up. We do the best we can. We aim for perfection in the hopes of achieving excellence. The same is true with this. We shall do the best we can. Then, we shall see.

Mental health has suffered, become tremendously more difficult to achieve, and even harder to maintain, since the advent of social media. Social media is literally starting to destroy the wellbeing of the minds of our children and all other users of social media. When people spend most of their time concentrating on digital platforms, it generally means that they are avoiding responsibility and inhibiting the ability of everyone else to advance as an organized, civilized society. The fears people had over particular video games and social networking have unfortunately become true for many reasons. Purportedly, investigations originally said that social media and various video games would not have a negative social impact; however, as with all technology and life, there has been a mixed bag.

For some people, social media has become its own form of a mental health crisis. Social media is often just a form of a mathematical calculation that creates content based on previous time spent online in concern to various activities and other personal interests. The reinforcement of the algorithm may lead people to believe that false or, at best, limited information is authentic when it may not be at all. This often seems to be the truth for many people when, in reality, much of social media is simply a marketing tool created to fit the expectations of what is wanted in order to sell merchandise to people who shop frequently online on the internet. Unfortunately, the algorithm brings content that the individual wants and has previously demonstrated a proclivity for, rather than content that is inherently honest or even healthy for the individual. This can lead to people creating and believing in a false manifestation of reality.

Social media is not truly understood by most people, as it is driven by an algorithm, and most people do not exactly understand what that concept entails or means. A simple to understand example would be if a person likes tan colored chairs and has searched for them previously online. Based on the amount of information the person will then receive afterwards about tan colored chairs, it is possible that the person is going to think everyone in the world likes tan colored chairs. This is especially true after a long duration of time occurs, because, after a while, there will be many things associated with tan colored chairs that are suggested by the algorithm. In reality, this is simply the case because at some point the person said they like tan colored chairs, not because everyone else likes tan colored chairs or even likes those types of chairs. The algorithm keeps reinforcing the microcosm of the reality the person has previously created. That is not truth; in fact, that is the limitation of information, which obviously prevents the assimilation of vast amounts of viewpoints. This leads to the inability to see things clearly and promotes bias or a false belief that bias may exist where it does not, even about tan colored chairs, let alone anything else in life.

Although neglectful parenting is part of the problem in some cases where technology has become a babysitter instead of the parents, it is not always the problem, either. It is important to spend time with children as parents. Time not being shared can be time spent by children searching for reality and care in areas where care and reality are not found and, even worse, predators may be. Guidance from a trusted elder promotes and provides confidence, emotional wellbeing, wisdom, physical security and helps tremendously in forming healthy relationships with other people over a lifetime.

No one should ever be ghosted, as the concept is horrible for multiple reasons. The trauma could be so significant that it has a never-ending negative effect on the person being purposely neglected permanently. We all are regal animals, and being purposely discarded like garbage is an unfair way for someone to have power over someone else. Ironically, it is also done most often by the people who act like refuse themselves. They are often the people who are the trash that needs to be discarded. The pain and abuse they purposely create serve as a mask generally to cover their own fear, insecurities and inabilities. The people who behave in such a manner frequently often feel powerless in life, and this manifests as a desire to have control over and dictate the actions of other people instead of searching for health within themselves. Sometimes, it is easier for people to blame others than accept their own foibles. This is not always the case when someone ends a relationship, but communication as to why a relationship is ending and will not continue is something that is healthy for all parties. Not doing so may cause irreparable harm to the other person.

People like to choose favorites among soft drinks, various sporting techniques and teams, what theatrical engagements they consider the most important, and sometimes they will even propagate a favorite restaurant, such as a fast-food venue, as part of their own independent makeup of how they view themselves. Usually, the cause of this behavior is a wantonness to belong to society, and this conduct can even be a display of desired power. This can play a role in how they construct their understanding of the world and even preclude them from being receptive to creative new thought processes. Sometimes this can lead to an inability to be receptive to new ideas and presentations. The truth is useful to all of us in having the ability to discover the person we want ourselves to be. The reality is that all these different options are important to have, as everyone's diversity provides opportunities in the complexity of the congregating community so that a multiplicity of options of thought provides the basis of availability for all people to be one while still being unique individuals. The truth is that all of the above is an exceptionally powerful experience and useful expression for all of us.

The reality is that all of the above choices are beneficial, as diversity is helpful for understanding. This is not just important for understanding other people, as the concept is even more vital for comprehending ourselves. People purposely take a favorable approach to learning when they know it advances their opportunities. This is something that is frequently perceived by the individual as being how to belong to something like a society or even civil society. We are allowed to search for a place of belonging. Sometimes, this will be a healthy endeavor; conversely, at other times, this action may be directed by a fear of not belonging to the society and village that surrounds us. Oftentimes, however, the reality is that this is a feature of a society created by people maintaining control and power by propagating a lack of power over the multitudes of citizens. Power is often a self-destructive illusion, too; be careful of the type of society you are so anxious to join; make sure it is truly positive and healthy. Maturing as an individual should involve love, not hate.

People often purposely pick a favorite to fit into a place of belonging, sometimes directed by a fear of not believing they belong anywhere, to anyone, at any time. Morals permit space for growth and are easy for us to adopt as principles of a core covenant of behavior to increase positivity in our own lives, neighborhoods and overall community as a whole. So, stop being judgmental; it only means you are afraid of being the one judged. Instead of speeding nowhere fast, pump the brakes, have unlimited opportunities available for the rest of your life, and enjoy the rest of your time. The other side of this concept also holds true though, too; being rebellious to the point of being decadent can cause societal decay.

Humans are like books: never judge any of them by their cover; you never know what is underneath. If you are not educated to make mental health assessments and judgments on care, you should not be asserting mental health labels on other people. Even many licensed professionals should not, as some are not truly honest with themselves either. Rigorous retraining may be necessary for our mental health professionals. We all need gentle kindness in our lives with ourselves and each other. Assumptions are often incorrect, and since we all can speak doofus fluently at any given time, we should refrain from being judgmental and making assumptions whenever we are capable of doing so.

Sometimes people blame other things for things they cannot control. We often assume that we understand the emergence of feelings and emotions that will and do arise in our lives. At certain times, we do, and at other times, we may never know if we are seeing things clearly. At best, we may only catch the gist of what has actually happened, the honesty behind the development of thoughts that occur, and the depth to which they are truly felt. We may never have the true knowledge of what those feelings or moments were like for another person. It is important to realize that this is true for all of us before we contemplate judging the consequences of emotion felt by other people. We may be able to be in a set of shoes for a moment; however, that does not mean we truly know what walking the path really feels like. Taking the time to truly listen is important and yet still may not provide insight.

The building blocks of life are designed to assist us when we are older after developing while we are younger and play a role in our evolution while making significant contributions to our decision-making process. Experience has a large impact on how we view life and the choices we make as we age. Later in life, when we are upset, many people do not realize that the same things that made them upset as individuals are the same issues that may have affected them emotionally as infants. When we need to perform basic human bodily functions, such as defecating, or urinating or when we are hungry, these things may all have a deleterious effect on our intelligence and decision-making. Sometimes it is best to remove an immediate impediment that may prohibit the ability for proper introspection. Not doing so may prevent us from using the wisdom gained from experience before deciding conclusively on a matter of substantial consequence that may impact on the future.

When we give in to our fearful thoughts, we are prone to make errors and, even worse, make a bad decision that costs us a lot of the good decisions we have made to get to that point in life. We are allowed to feel the vulnerability that naturally is adjoined to our own existence. As such, it is important to remember that truth is a matter of acceptance and accountability, never force. It is important to accept truth on the merits of it being what it is, not what we want or would like it to be. Finding truth is the process of just simply accepting the actuality of something for what it accurately is in reality. Even then, we may be incapable in the moment of being able to see the entire truth clearly.

Nonverbal communication with those on the autism spectrum seems to be far more effective and less overwhelming for the autistic person. This is often true for all people when they are overly inundated with a case of sensory overload from too much stimulation being provided by sources, especially multiple sources simultaneously. Even the most altruistic of help becomes threatening and imposing when everything starts to blend together into a garbled mess that is reminiscent of a Charlie Brown teacher's voice, where everything sounds distorted and the same, which results when the mind is overstimulated.

People are not just individual; they are situational as well. Like patience, controlling our own opportunities when impulsivity control may be difficult is made even harder when temptation and allure are offered in addition to those moments of enticement. It is necessary to have discipline and to maintain self-control if someone is attempting to achieve something of great importance. Think for yourself, as it is a necessary resource in situations that inherently require critical reasoning skills. No matter what, the day always resolves into the twilight of our own recesses of our own minds, bodies and souls.

Getting things done right the first time matters. Measure twice, cut once. Double checking is a wonderful practice to incorporate into all of our lives with each and everything we do, even the seemingly menial tasks. Double and even triple checking can reduce stress levels instantaneously during a moment of self-doubt and instill confidence later, especially if things go awry. Double checking also saves time from making mistakes. Having to go back and do things a second time can be difficult, and it can cost time and money. Double checking is an effective, simple preventive measure of stress reduction. Double checking can also instill a sense of assurance in being prepared for important situations.

Facing each other can be exceptionally difficult, and escalating tensions can be very hard to overcome; however, facing ourselves is an even harder task and one less likely to be initiated. The people who are unable or unwilling to face themselves are often the first ones to cast aspersions on other people. When there are situations of negativity, most people look at everything and everyone else before taking the time to examine the situation honestly. When everyone else on the road is bad at driving, it is often easier not to look in the mirror and see who the bad driver really is.

The health difficulties faced by the male and female genders are sometimes the same; however, they can also be very different physically and mentally as well. In reality, everyone is an individual, and their development is completely their own and only true to them. This is true with the psychological evolution for all of us as well. While there do seem to be some characteristics that are inherently true for all of us, things such as responses, choices made previously, and even the nature and nurture of each individual's upbringing are likely to have an impact on why we may act or react differently in a given situation. Due to this, the long-term trauma and prevalence of post-traumatic stress disorders are likely to have dire long-term health consequences for any individual who has been placed in negative situations at any age, especially, if during their youth and particularly, if for a long duration.

When people are discussing the Oedipal complex, what they are really discussing is the Electra complex. At the time Sigmund Freud started the practice that has now become what is referred to as psychology, it was difficult to find people to sit on a couch and talk about their feelings. While Dr. Freud did have some male patients, his patients were initially mostly female because, for various reasons, most men were employed and females were not. The problem came for Freud when he attempted to get published. At the time, women had not yet received equal rights anywhere in the civilized world, and, as such, no one was very interested in reading about what women were concerned about or their thoughts. Even most romantic authors' works were written by men like Chaucer and Shakespeare to that point in history. To get published, Freud changed the subjects in his writings to be about males, even though many of his initial findings were from women. It would be Freud's contemporary, Carl Jung, who would first mention the concept of the Electra complex in 1913. To this day, what is thought of as the Oedipal complex most likely is the Electra complex.

There seems to be an escalating portion of society that has become more prevalent and that has caused most communities to be dealing with an increased lack of decency. Dignity and ethics were taken for granted in years gone by.

While many men have been known to engage in such negative behavior, it also now appears as though key, strong, instrumental women often bully other women only to display power. Unfortunately, this has become a part of the culture, and due to the commonality of manipulation, bullying and even criminality, these behaviors have become more acceptable as daily occurrences in theory, while obviously detrimental to all people in reality. A person's personal proclivities should never be forced upon anyone else in concern to certain intimate individual interests.

Physical actions have been proven to release positive endorphins that help to reduce stress, in addition to physicality promoting a healthier lifestyle. Faith in a higher entity also has been shown to be a useful and successful methodology for obtaining clarity, balance and peace of mind. This is demonstrated in many ways when people attend religious functions without even knowing it. For instance, getting up and down repeatedly in church gets the positive endorphins kicking in with a form of minimal exercise, which helps to promote health while subconsciously making people feel better. A general feeling of being healthier is also accomplished by being given a wafer to eat as nourishment for the soul and the physical body. Participating in spiritual endeavors can literally and figuratively help to improve someone's mental state and promote a healthier environment for every person who participates. Positivity is also found in being part of a positive group dynamic that encourages healthy discourse, promotes taking personal responsibility and highlights community.

We are all essential. That word, essential, is a good example of the do-gooders meaning well and doing us all in during the process. While it was surely interesting for all of us during the Covid epidemic, there was also a large degree of pressure, stress and strain placed upon everyone as well.xiv We were separated and sometimes felt cut off. Those things that we endeavor to do and the people that we love and choose to be around for health, pleasure, relaxation and comfort were all taken away for substantial periods of time. Even worse, there were sometimes situations where people were not allowed to be there for individuals, comfort the ones they loved or say goodbye to them in person as they died. All of this because people were acting responsibly in their concern for themselves and one another. The stress then and the post-traumatic aftereffects from those Covid incarcerations have led many to believe, unfortunately, that they are not essential. The truth is that everyone alive right now is essential. All lives are essential. All life is essential. Knowing that each of our lives is essential is in itself essential. We are all all essential, as are the animals and the planet Earth.

The aftermath of Covid has presented many psychological concerns for adults and children. Post-traumatic stress disorders from a multitude of realities of those years need to be addressed, from the word essential being used to empower some and minimize others during Covid to the effects left behind by not having normal social integration in regard to our youth. Not being able to attend certain functions like school daily will have a certain effect on some people, while not being able to attend graduations, funerals or even be in the hospital when a loved one was dying will influence society for generations to come. The damage that has been inflicted already has left people feeling lost. It has created a sense where, instead of investigating the truth, people tend to pronounce their viewpoint as fact.

Often, in our current environment, it feels as though people try to exert force as if doing so will change the truth surrounding an item, circumstance or an understanding of reality. Truth is always a matter of acceptance, never force. Cleopatra would espouse the simple reality that the truth will always emerge no matter how deep a person attempts to dive into and submerge themselves in the river of denial. Mental health assessments could be based on observing a lack of maturity established in actions by fully grown adults as they attempt to ignore basic teaching lessons that many people ascertain during preschool or early grade school. If the objects and wholes being used are and remain the same size, then attempting to fit a square peg into a whole shaped like a circle or attempting to fit a circle into a whole shaped like a square does not work. Many people spend most of their lives attempting to figure out that they are incapable of influencing an outcome that is different from what they want. Most of the time, they will spend their energy focusing on forcing an objective or an item to be different than what they know it is in relation to the truth, reality and its original intentions for why it was created.

On the other hand, life is enigmatic, and the impossible of today is sometimes the reality of tomorrow. After investigation, life is sometimes scrutable. In unique cases, remarkable and outstanding results are obtainable when will is demonstrated in a special manner. When an individual or a group steps up and refuses to lose, pledging to never give up, ever, no matter how difficult the opportunity may be to achieve, it is incredible how accomplishments may be obtained when the final objective becomes a tangible finished product. The ability to compartmentalize and see how things are and be able to associate seemingly disparate, disjointed items with an appropriate aptitude applied that brings these ideas together is a necessary component for deciphering what is real and obtainable and what may be only theoretical. Understanding limitations, recognizing boundaries, and accepting truth are always inherent necessary components for finding success with even the simplest of endeavors. Most of life is beyond our control, and seeing clearly what we can and cannot do is always a benefit. Science being intertwined with brilliance, education, and observation being utilized by kind, caring, and considerate therapists is the future of mental health care.

The study of mental health must be improved dramatically. Due to the lack of integration of neurological studies, physical studies into each person's central nervous system, and the coincidences that are often considered to be groundbreaking psychological diagnoses and significant in the field for further examination and exploration, although they have never been proven consistently or conclusively, it is necessary to state the obvious that all three fields, while maybe not pseudo sciences, are at best fields of inquiry that are still in their infancy period as true fields of investigation, let alone as fields of medical comprehension or understanding that are on par with the rest of the medical community.

How is a human being defined as normal? Are baseline studies done on chemicals, bacteria, and balances in the brain, starting from infancy onward, as they are in all other fields of medicine? Much as each person's heart is physically in a different location within the chest cavity, is it possible to conclude that people have varying homeostatic levels of functional necessities to be able to maneuver their way through what is a different landscape for each and every human being in the course of normal life? Are we able to see normal conditions of cognitive functioning and be able to appreciate the circumstances that may alter the aftereffects of significant impact, especially physical or mental trauma? Is someone mentally impaired if they believe they are able to assist another person with mental or physical health? Would you consider someone mentally imbalanced if they cried in public? How about if it was later determined that they cried in public on the anniversary of when they lost a parent, friend, significant other, or especially one of their children? Who, in their relationships, has had total tranquility at all moments at all times without any sense of feeling alone or desperately trying to maintain a sense of stability and care in difficult situations? Who knows the exact chemical balances of their brain and how it is functioning at this exact moment? Do impacts on a person's spine and other portions of the brain stem mean that they may never recover from their condition and that they are permanently damaged in all instances, both physically and mentally?

There are wonderful health care professionals who are altruistic, thorough, and caring in their field of professional endeavor. Yet we also have people who profess to be doctors, physicians, life coaches, and other members of the health care field who talk about the stories of patients to others with a pompous attitude. Sometimes these are very highly regarded medical professionals; however, many of them are often so-so at best in the care they provide. These people are typically more about style than substance in many facets of their own lives and are quite regularly judgmental without having the proper requisite information to make an informed decision. In fact, there is an arrogant attitude frequently presented by some people in the health care field in concern to other members of the health care field who are less qualified. There are also those people who are less qualified in the medical industry who are quick to dismiss accredited individuals, companies, and fields of medicine for not having a valid purpose in reality for how these entities conduct their business. On the surface, there is almost an indication that these people in the health care field have achieved more or know something better than the rest of the population in relation to their mental and physical activities. This is seen far too frequently in many health care fields nowadays. This is especially true with psychiatrists and psychologists. There are way too many lives that are being influenced by mental health professionals claiming to be experts who may need skilled assistance and good guidance themselves. If cerebral accomplishments involve mental acuity, then are not these the first people who should suggest sincerely that further investigation into the fields of neuroscience, physical studies of the body, including of the central nervous system, and psychological observations should be part of the same fields of inquiry, and treatment should be completely independent of assessment and assumptions based on other human beings? It seems these fields are filled with narcissism, ego, and, unfortunately, even predators who seek to fill a void within themselves. Complete research and retraining may be necessary for many health care providers in these supposed fields of expertise immediately. Until a comprehensive understanding has been achieved of how the three seemingly disparate fields of neuroscience, central nervous function and more individualized psychological care models are integrated, there are significant deficiencies in these fields of study. The combination of medical data should help avoid erroneous judgments, false prognoses and should also help to prevent severe mental degeneration.

It will one day be possible to understand the science and medical practice of psychology and turn it into a part of real mainstream health care; however, that is not the truth now. With the way psychology is currently structured, there are too many independent variables that promote wrongful diagnoses and misinterpretations for emergency care, immediate care, follow up care, and aftercare models for providing therapy. The current evaluation system is severely limited by the patient's ability to articulate what may be wrong and by the doctor's own proclivity toward the formation of bias due to his or her own experiences, agenda, and possibly his or her ego as well. Even just not hearing something correctly may alter a care path tremendously. A simple thing like being hungry, having to go to the bathroom, or feeling pressure due to a multitude of conceivable correlating considerations may lead to a false manifestation of reality or at least alter the ability to perceive at any time in all contexts. This is true for both patients and doctors.

Brain studies in the field of mental health will be aided by nanotechnology in the future through the ability to map each individual's brain function from birth. As the person grows to maturity, the synaptic functions, as well as normal chemical balances and blood flows, will be monitored nonstop. When the neural pathways set, the individual's personal normal homeostatic levels will be able to be monitored and noted. If there is any type of trauma or a form of cognitive degeneration as the patient becomes older, it will be instantly recognizable to the doctor, administrative staff and all future caregivers. With new advents into the field of preventive and preemptive health care, the patient will be able to monitor the state of their mental and physical health with home monitoring devices.

Many neurologists are concerned that impairments in cognitive function are being over diagnosed by many of their fellow doctors from all fields. There seems to be a surplus of patients who are hypochondriacs searching for something to be wrong with them as individuals and for procedures to be performed, even if inappropriate. Unfortunately, what is occurring is that the patients often search for doctors until they find one willing to perform completely unnecessary surgeries for the most part, if not just totally unjustifiable surgeries altogether. A hypochondriac should not be dictating their own care, especially to the point they are finding medical professionals to assist them in causing themselves harm. Hysteria by the patient should not dictate care considerations of future health care implementations. Reasonable, educated, common sense practices should always prevail. Doctors in the future will have instantaneous access to information about the mental state of the patient from all prior at-home readings even before beginning an in-office exam. This should help to distinguish between real concerns and those that may need other support.

For a health care professional, it is always important to be thorough with a patient. This begins by asking the patient how he or she feels. It then continues by palpating the patient for any possible physical warning signs of disease while listening to the patient and by doing a complete investigation into all information that can be accumulated, including hereditary predispositions and any preexisting conditions. Combining the information collected from directly interviewing the patient during counseling while also having full contextual knowledge of how the patient's brain functions should help lead to a more exact diagnosis with a higher probability of a successful prognosis. Also, any type of alteration in brain chemical function may be observed more quickly. This may take time, as failure is often a necessary step to successfully finding a path to being able to truly provide a patient's consciousness with a pathway and an opportunity for the patient's conscious behavior to reach its full potential with, hopefully, a newfound clarity of respect for themselves and all other individuals. It is also important to note that rushing to judgment and assuming something is only a psychosomatic response may be tantamount to malfeasance if it turns out that there is an underlying neurological disturbance that may be a temporary complication or be an unforeseen cause that perchance may be life threatening.

Barbaric treatments such as lobotomies and electric shock were once encouraged and looked upon favorably by intelligent people in the field of health care. Scientists were aware of electrical impulses in the brain and yet may not have had the cognition themselves to realize they were not firing on the right synaptic frequencies. In many cases, these vicious methodologies of supposed care created more impediments than they helped to alleviate. Today's model of care can be tomorrow's cause for concern and dismay for many patients. As many doctors have hypothesized, is it possible that the coronavirus vaccine that was used is tied to the alarming number of current cases of cardiomyopathy effecting the muscles and heart of many young men? Did the vaccine cause or exacerbate underlying neuropathies or other neurological conditions in many patients? Should this possibility be combined with vaccine studies to determine the probability of potential long-term effects?

Many people with tattoos regret getting them for a multitude of reasons later on in life. Tattoo removal is an incredibly painful experience that has become more commonplace over the past couple of decades. Tattoos may be favorable to some people; however, all tattoos become permanent timestamps that come with both positive and negative consequences. While a tattoo may help one to honor and remember, it may also prove to be detrimental in attempting to move forward in life. A tattoo can become an impediment to growth as it transforms into a constant symbol from the past and does not allow for a future that is independent in thought and action from the permanent reminder. Doctors used to view tattoos as one of the first signs of mental disease, as tattoos, by nature, are a form of human disfigurement and self-mutilation. While they are more commonplace today, they often still accompany people with various mental disease diagnoses on a frequent basis. The same reasoning applies when a person participates in branding themselves.

When a stroke patient needs care after the incident, this is one of the rare times in the current health care setting when studies into the patient's central nervous system, psychological wellbeing, and neurological functions are combined with the patient's need for physical therapy to determine health and aid in recovery. This concept of a care model should be more commonplace and leads to a general notion that baseline studies need to be done thoroughly throughout a person's lifespan. This type of care should not be performed only on a reactionary basis after a patient has gone through such a difficult medical diagnosis. Improvements to baseline data studies that correlate a patient's individual information with general precursors established from material collected from the majority of people who have previously suffered a stroke, may lead to the ability to help halt the onset of a stroke in the future.

The final frontiers facing us are space, the human mind and our oceans. We need an emphasis reminiscent of NASA, the National Aeronautics and Space Administration, in regard to the exploration of our oceans, and this type of thorough examination is necessary with our brains, too. The planet is seventy one percent oceans and seas. It is estimated that over eighty percent of Earth's oceans and seas remain unexamined. It is surprising that we know so little about the majority of our own planet. While people say we know more about space than about our oceans, this is not necessarily true, as, in reality, in outer space there are at least one hundred billion different galaxies, with each galaxy containing one hundred billion stars. The truth is we know even less about the human brain, and it needs more exploration as well.

The environmental learning centers we will be creating and initiating as a part of this new health care policy will be a basis for creating such exploration. We will work our way to learn the truth about our oceans, soil, and atmospheric conditions in a manner that will promote a healthier environment for all inhabitants of our planet Earth. The environmental learning centers will also help with space exploration as well, as they will serve as a template for how human beings will have to be able to adapt to different atmospheric conditions, soil situations, and water needs on other planets if we are going to be able to inhabit other planets in the future. The environmental learning centers will provide training grounds for how to find ways for us to survive initially and thrive eventually while establishing similar constructions of environmental learning centers when we first begin to live on other planets in the future. In reality, while aiding humans, these Earth based environmental learning centers are also truly the space exploration learning centers we will need in order to exist in the future. Creating and even living in these centers, especially initially, will test our mental capabilities, require us to increase our intelligence and fortify our psychological resolve. These centers will require further investigation into ourselves as human beings in totality. This will include supplementary studies into our physical and mental wellbeing and aid in the application of medicine across a plethora of fields, enhancing all life capabilities.

The most elusive system in the history of medicine within the human body is the brain and how it correlates with our ability to survive and function throughout the course of a person's lifetime. We need to proceed from our current elementary education in the understanding of brain function to explore the vast depths of potential, so we may finally unlock the powers that are super that are hidden within each and every person. Also, in the interim, it is believed that the number of misdiagnosed cases concerning cranial function is extremely extensive, and, meanwhile, the care being provided is exceptionally expensive. The time has come when using mathematical data from history may help to formulate patterns of prevention that deter the likelihood of a catastrophic life altering situation for all people. Baseline data studies will help to create improvements by correlating information as to the normal equilibrium for each individual, so the best level of care is possible and adhered to. The investigation into our brains will ignite our capabilities.

The truth is, we are all essential. We all have pain, and we all know sorrow. Happiness awaits us if we overcome ourselves. Our salvation will be found in the mercy we create for ourselves and all others. The possibilities to augment all of life are here, and the time to pursue these endeavors is now. Every person has significant value. Even the dumbest person on Earth probably knows something that the smartest person on Earth does not. Everyone needs a hug and love. Live, laugh, love and remember, practice makes perfect.

CHAPTER 6

INSURANCE

Family is the cornerstone that gives shape to our existence. Family first, always, no matter what. Family first, no matter what, is care first, no matter what. Family are the people you care about. Family plans for health insurance will be designed to be independent for each family. Plans will be adaptable, so each individual member of a family is capable of finding proper coverage for their health care necessities and possible needs with choices available. Being a family member will be defined by statute as pertaining only to parents, their children, and any other dependents who meet eligibility requirements. Cost effective measures for pursuing individual care needs for each family member's specific health care needs will be available. These coverages will be part of plans covered by the individual health plan described and provided by different health plan insurance companies doing business in each distinct health plan coverage area while providing national coverage. From state to state, these companies will be providing all necessary policies through options on various tiers with procedures in accordance with all pertinent individual state statutes as well as national standards. All procedures necessary due to precautions will be followed in accordance with all applicable laws and regulations, too. While companies will be permitted and encouraged to cross state lines for competi-

tion in the marketplace to help lower prices for people, the statutes for each state must be independently recognized. It is time for stolat for all in any language: 100 years of good health for everyone.

All means all. The time to begin is now. The sooner we commence implementation, the better. We will work to progress quality time to exist immediately for as many as possible. The layers and textures needed to move forward will be addressed appropriately when timing is optimal for additional implementation. Optimal performance means prime accurate coordination excellence. The immediate implementation of this program will help all people of all ages everywhere it applies. Hopefully, our future will provide an opportunity for an existence with less pain and suffering for all people of all ages, including today's young people; our investment in them may pay dividends and benefits beyond mere hope.

It is important that we understand that implementing actions rather than words is a matter of necessity, that earning success builds confidence and creates courage for future goals and pursuits to be accomplished. Sooner than later, this new plan of action will be recognized as an important step forward that permits every one of us to feel good, literally and metaphorically. Growth and education keep us young. Initiating this program is an oath for us to start an enrichment of life on all fronts in an environment of positivity for all moving forward for a very long time while producing new innovations as well as stimulating generations of massive growth opportunities for the foreseeable future and beyond without any limitations.

Affordable, convenient health care that is available with total customization is a necessity for all people. While some would question the importance of insurance being the first domino in a logical sequence of progression that leads to the meaning of life for each of us and all of us, the reality is that implementing the insurance change discussed here really is that hearthstone. The insurance industry is in all aspects of everything throughout the entire world around us, and due to this, there is already a large amount of international and domestic insurance communication all over the world.

Health care needs to change dramatically and quickly. How will we react on a national level? How will we go forward with other nations? We need to tailor our energies to the realities of our environment. Care is compassion with an appropriate, affordable level of insurance coverage with respect to the individual as part of a healthy environment for everyone. Being healthy means being sound in mind, body and soul. These are issues of paramount importance today and forever.

Where we are going should be looked at like trying to find our way through a maze. With mazes, the best way to find the path you are looking for is not to start at the beginning and try to find a way to the end; the best way to deal with a maze is to start at the end and then find the path to the beginning and, with some mazes, even the path of least resistance. Many people refer to this methodology now as reverse engineering. Reverse engineering is knowing the expected result as to what is being created and then working backwards to find a way to make that result happen in reality on a repeatable basis consistently. We are not reinventing the wheel, just using base systems that were

provided and implementing new concepts such as artificial intelligence to permit immediate exponential growth. If we need to adjust, we shall do so and then achieve our goals accordingly.

Most people seem to like the idea of a doctor who knows you for most of your life. Many people alive now grew up in a time and age when their expectation was probably that the doctor they knew when they were younger may be the person trusted as their doctor for the rest of that patient's life, or at least long term. While those wholesome days of yesteryear may not be doable in the here and now, the application of the process described in this section will work effectively to mimic that ideal as close as possible. It will entail the need for governments to work closely with insurance companies and institutions of financial consideration, as well as pharmaceutical industry experts, regarding what requirements and considerations need to be accomplished to make sure we have all things prepared for success on all levels and for all possible consequences for all people.

Under the Affordable Care Act, there is a truly unfortunate reality for all. There are large price differences between the care you can receive locally and if you want to travel anywhere else. Out of market costs under the current structure serve to limit freedom far worse than accessibility to insurance does. This means that the Affordable Care Act is providing a disservice as an overall solution to the needs of the people in the situation of public health and the ability to be as healthy as possible. Out of market costs prohibit freedom of movement from place to place for most individuals currently.

As many people are already aware, the Northeast of the United States of America is a geographic location where there are many small states that are all within a few hours' drive of one another. It is possible to drive through Maine, New Hampshire, Vermont, Massachusetts, Connecticut, and Rhode Island within a few hours and even have time to make it outside of New England in the same day to New York, New Jersey and Pennsylvania. The following reality based situation is one concrete example of how the Affordable Care Act, the ACA, actually hurts people as it restricts geographic movement with financial risk.

Right now, if a family were going to see the leaves change colors in any state in New England and that family left the state in which they live to travel to a different state, and something unfortunate accidentally occurred and members of the family needed medical attention, especially if hospitalization were required, that family would immediately find out how unfriendly the current situation for individuals is when it comes to the cost of hospitalization and all the things patients must face in using their individual insurance when it comes to health care. Most insurance policies currently have an out-of-pocket maximum that is two and a half times higher for out-of-network occurrences than the costs are for in-network incidences. For example, a family's in-state out-of-pocket maximum in-network could be $20,000; however, that exact same occurrence with the exact same care provided out of state could immediately reach an out-of-network out-of-pocket maximum of $50,000. In addition, the current level of health care insurance leads to hit or miss care. That is not good for customers who need emergency services, let alone doctors. The reality is that any state in the United States of America could be used for the preceding example of how an increase in financial risk can negate freedom. Amazing affordable care anywhere and at all times is what anyone would really want.

The importance of improvements with artificial intelligence forecast modeling is demonstrated by cost variance for the consumer. Take someone with preexisting conditions; the artificial intelligence should help that consumer to budget appropriately with prior knowledge, utilizing individual forecast modeling to also provide especially good predictions that permit each participant to prepare to properly select health care coverage on various tiers and with various options that fit best. This will include all possibilities the artificial intelligence predictive modeling is capable of for the individual, as that person may see either improvement or the possible occurrence of a condition that requires more coverage throughout the year via insurance or with pharmaceutical assistance. Not every circumstance is predictable; however, modeling will help. We will include all people who are infirm. There will be no denial of insurance for preexisting conditions. All means all.

When in need as a patient, the consumer will have shockingly low-priced same day repair with maximized emergency care available and a sense of affordability that provides optimism that the associated costs will not be debilitating to survival. Instead, much as with the necessary emergency care, each person will have coverage that hopefully provides relief.

Right now, there are managers at major big box department stores, including young minority women, who cannot afford insurance through the state or their jobs. Employees are being offered the chance to work thirty hours a week, and not thirty-two hours, so they will not qualify for group health care with their companies. Often, the cost of an individual health insurance plan is too high to afford with the current wages they are being paid. If these young ladies are not being offered the opportunity to afford health care coverage, it is safe to assume that the entire marketplace of all potential consumers is being affected, as we will all eventually be patients at some point in our lives. Being able to afford health insurance is necessary for all people.

The government subsidies currently given as tax credits for each state to lower the cost of insurance should be given directly to the people. Each person should be awarded an amount that can only be used for health care in a health savings account program. This is needed because, otherwise, uninsured people showing up at emergency rooms can cause an unexpected burden on insurance companies, pharmaceutical companies, the state, and, most importantly, the people of the state. When the state has unexpected losses, it is the taxpayers from those states who feel the burden with increased taxes and reductions in public programs. Unforeseen losses negatively impact the future viability of costs too. If a person does not accept insurance or does not engage in purchasing a program in the future and then uses an emergency medical care facility while receiving that care for free today, then that person will lose the amount received today in the future with reduced stipends so as not to unfairly burden the remainder of the collective of society. People on group insurance will receive less aid as the cost of their programs on group insurance is usually far less expensive. If that person reenters the workplace without group insurance available, then they will be reevaluated, and a full individual stipend will apply. Pertinent period prorations may need to be calculated in each of these situations.

Native Americans and all soldiers, known or unknown, after discharge, need to have access to excellent health care for the rest of their lives. They earned it. For instance, if there were a ten level tiered system of concierge health insurance where level one is basic care and level ten is on a right to try consideration level for those facing the most serious of imminent health crises, then level four would be extended for all military veterans in a long overdue thank you for all soldiers, and the same level program of level four would be extended to all Native Americans in a longer overdue thank you. Other applications can be determined on a state-by-state basis.

The provisions extended to military personnel are only meant to be augmentations to the current military model, as some veterans do receive excellent coverage already. The same would be true for all Native American health care programs as well, as it would only serve to augment if there is a system that works well already for the majority of each tribal population. Each tribe should be able to make up their own minds on what system would work best for each tribe's indigenous people. The point here is to help further, not to reinvent the wheel by replacing a system that works for the majority of people it helps already. If an item of care needs attention, though, this is the time to get it right. In addition, veterans' rides to all health facilities would be covered by insurance, and this will include known and unknown soldiers and shall be covered in full by insurance always. It once took the Society of the Cincinnati to provide for our soldiers after the Revolutionary War; action is needed again.

All former military personnel should have access, after being honorably discharged, to a level of care similar to what they had while they were active members of the United States military services, whether their actions and involvement be known or unknown. As such, from this point forward, all soldiers and, in this vein, all of those who have never even been recognized will be awarded a good tier of coverage automatically after a period of time, and it will be enhanced for those who have committed more time in appreciation for their service to freedom in a long overdue thank you for their actions. Again, all Native Americans, as all Americans need good health care, will also qualify in a longer overdue thank you as well.

Holistic and homeopathic remedies will be available through certain programs offered on all tiers via a la carte options and through additional rider coverage if requested. This will be done as necessary so that creative options on how to formulate the right plan for each family and person can be met easily. Holistic homeopathic medication pharmaceutical coverage options will be included in a range of treatments from basic needs to invasive right to try levels while being offered within tiered concierge service programs. Individual necessities will be met by a multitude of variant holistic options within each tier and with varying pharmaceutical possibilities too. When it comes to medications being administered, people will have the option to start with the least invasive remedy to begin with on all levels and then have access to other medications of more severity that usually have more side effects as well, administered appropriately in a step-by-step progression model of care.

Formularies used by the pharmaceutical industry can differ from plan to plan and on various tiers for a variety of cost effective measures that should be quantified a year in advance so any consideration necessary for the consumption of any medication can be planned in advance by any person purchasing a prescribed medication so as to know what program they should take advantage of in the purchase of any pharmaceutical program attached to their insurance coverage for the following year. This should also provide a quite lucrative marketplace for the pharmaceutical companies involved in the manufacturing of prescription medicines that will be part of the insurance industry programs moving forward.

Right to try will be available directly through big pharma on this tiered system so that profit margins will improve significantly for all pharmaceutical companies in the marketplace as well as the insurance companies. Pharma will be receiving its money directly as always. Research and development is where most of this money is collected currently for pharma companies. The new systems approach should provide a platform for much higher financial yield moving forward in the foreseeable future, and projections should be forecasted to increase exponentially. Right to try levels will not have caps financially and will be what the market will bear and is capable of providing in a state-by-state initiative.

Discount pharmacy possibilities may be a way of deferring some costs for some people as well and could be owned by the health care companies. This would be especially beneficial for patients who are taking medications that have no generic counterpart. Drug prices can become prohibitive when there is no alternative medication or a cost-effective substitute that exists in a generic form. Specific options on various tiers may provide a more balanced financial reality than some people face now. It would be a helpful time saver for pharmacies and patients to have coupons from certain sites and those that are directly from the manufacturer streamlined by direct input to all pharmacies for billing purposes in advance.

New fields of study will include a multitude of different subjects and will also offer different models of care that can be included on each level and with varying a la carte options on each tier as well. Treatment services provided year-round generally tend to qualify for assistance more quickly than do services offered quarterly, so henceforth, all coverage will be applicable on an annual basis. Annual reviews will be necessitated for each occurrence.

There should be further research into the positive effects of black seed oil and other remedies that need to be explored further to understand their true relevance and potency in providing care. Such possible remedies may lead to much higher profit margins for pharma companies as well if associated properly with a new tiered system of coverage.

Universal family is not just a brotherhood or sisterhood, as women and men are the same in equality but different in their health care needs as all individuals are. Women should not be forced to face some charges that men do not, as men are not capable of giving birth organically from conception. As such, free delivery of all babies should be available for all women.

Ambulance fees should be included in all health care insurance programs. Transportation costs of all types should be refunded if the costs are associated with an emergency situation of dire need, too. Currently, emergency transportation appears to be a facet abused by many municipalities.

Weekly pharmaceutical delivery for the elderly, already parceled for daily use to avoid the potential for overdose, would be helpful, although the current procedures used need to be addressed. The packages need to be protected from tampering yet able to be opened by the elderly. Right now, many elderly people have difficulty opening their transported medications when delivered presorted. They are packaged as such to prevent the theft of illicit substances during transport. A happy medium seems possible with proper introspection.

Dietary needs are different for every individual and should be specific to the realities of each person's existence to promote the best health going forward. Investment in nutrition by consumers should also help lower exposure costs for insurance companies. A receipt-based program to reduce insurance costs may provide additional riders or tier choices for pharma, too. The long-term effects of a healthier society should theoretically mean less need for medical assistance in the short, interim and long term, too.

Physical therapy, rehabilitation, and other forms of outpatient treatment should be included as part of certain levels of available coverage plans on various tiers. Riders may also be available as well. Newly established treatment quality indicators, through which deficiencies are identified on a preemptive basis rather than waiting for deficits or defects to be recognized after a significant injury, should be included in some options as well. The ability to forecast deficiencies is likely to become more prevalent with artificial intelligence forecast modeling being utilized more often. There should also be constant reassessment for anyone disabled on a yearly basis, too, to see if they still meet disability criteria.

Greeters who help wheel patients into and out of the hospital as part of the patients' hospital stays and at health care facilities should be available for those in need of such assistance. Participation will be part of a courtesy community counseling program, which may be a way for students of all ages to earn financial compensation or gain educational credits in a degree program. Engaging the community with consideration by participating in programs that instill professional potential and confidence in our youth today will build our leadership population for the greater good of all societies tomorrow.

Dental, vision, and hearing care need to be included in basic health care insurance programs moving forward. If licensed professionals in these fields were permitted to give recommendations on health care necessities when a potential issue is first noticed, a large number of serious illnesses could be treated much earlier, leading to far better long-term results. The observation of certain precursors by vision, dental, and hearing specialists will help to prolong life by enabling symptoms to be treated before they become far worse problems if these professionals are included in the mainstream health care system.

Vision insurance works well, and companies should be inclined to maintain appropriate coverage as they are currently structured. The only difference would be its individual inclusion upon the purchase of appropriate coverage, where vision does not come with all levels available for coverage but is included in many different options with varying levels of coverage. Vision, hearing, and dental insurance may be provided through additional riders or in an a la carte fashion available on all tiers. Surgical tiers and options for consideration, such as retinal repairs, cataract removal, glaucoma, corneal transplants, and other common eye surgeries and ailments, should also remain available under necessary health insurance base coverage. LASIK, laser assisted in situ keratomileusis, should be made available either through the purchase of various options on different tiers or through the purchase of an additional rider. Additional research should be done into what contributes to wet and dry macular degeneration in order to see if any methods of preventing the onset of the debilitating eye issues can be found or if a cure may finally be discovered immediately.

An important caveat that does need correction with vision insurance is the ability to see your ophthalmologist at least once per year. Often, many programs currently offer availability for only one checkup every two years. The first diagnostic testing for any type of prescription for eyeglasses should also be covered in all plans, with aftercare dependent upon the tier and program chosen. Otherwise, the system of surgical needs as part of the base health care program and other vision coverage that is purchased separately through what is currently called the supplemental insurance marketplace should remain mostly the same. The only difference should be that supplemental coverage for further eyeglass testing and eyewear will be able to be purchased by each individual as additional coverage on a higher tier or still added as additional coverage a la carte, much as the system currently works.

From welding to computer glare, eye issues can be devastating to our ability to perform our daily tasks. It is hard to do anything when you cannot see clearly. Styes may form, along with multiple other medical issues that can cause impediments. Diabetes, hypertension, certain forms of cancer such as melanoma, multiple sclerosis, and other autoimmune medical concerns are examples of very serious medical conditions for which eye doctors and specialists, such as ophthalmologists and optometrists, may be very helpful in making predictions that could lead to a preliminary diagnosis of these conditions and possibly other diseases as well, far ahead of when symptoms appear due to another severe phenomenon.

Recent findings suggest bacterial buildups within the body may be leading to different forms of cancer. Some bacteria are already recognized as carcinogens that play a major role in the onset of various forms of cancer. In addition, bacteria have also been shown to be a contributing factor in increasing the likelihood of damage to DNA. Also, other forms of bacteria may result in toxic metabolites. Helicobacter pylori is a bacterium that is a common cause of stomach ulcers and a contributing factor in stomach cancer. Bacteria such as E. coli and Fusobacterium nucleatum are often demonstrated to be associated with causing colorectal cancer. Is it possible that not brushing your teeth enough leads to bacterial growth that collects in a person's stomach and leads to stomach and maybe intestinal cancer, too? Do bacteria that build up orally from not brushing regularly exacerbate underlying situations that lead to issues, creating more opportunities for cancerous precursor conditions such as human papillomavirus? There also appears to be a link between oral hygiene and diabetes. This, as well as a possible link between oral hygiene and effects on the heart, should be examined immediately for long-term prognosis possibilities. Healthy smiles for kids and adults literally sometimes mean that a healthy smile indicates a person is truly healthy. Emergency dental care, including implants, is a necessary component to take into account when thinking about the relationship of individuals when it comes to the necessity of dental care and insurance coverage options available on higher tiers or via a rider. Consultations with dental doctors should be considered when restructuring the health care portfolio for all individuals.

Hearing is an often-overlooked component of health care that is obvious when you think about being deaf and trying to drive and not being able to hear the ambulance or fire truck behind you. Hearing loss can lead to feelings of anger, depression and even paranoia. When you do not hear people walking towards you and then they start talking to you, it can startle anyone at any given time. The necessary component of successful communication and conversation is good listening. Ear, nose and throat doctor coverage should be made available, and preliminary testing should be done to establish baselines for all individuals. Coverage for auditory specialists via choices on tiers and rider availability is also required.

While do no harm is not a good place to begin patient care for adults, children or to apply to healthy development, there does come a point in the Hippocratic Oath when do no harm becomes the best we can do for each patient's need for quality time while they face end-of-life decisions. Physician assistants and nurse practitioners will not have to worry about losing career opportunities; in fact, their altruistic nature will be more important than ever before. The ability to understand the situation and the needs of each individual patient facing environmental shifts and even end-of-life decisions is more vital than ever. These highly trained health care professionals will be the ones providing dignity and respect to those who have experienced life problems and need assistance. Hospice care will no longer be available; instead, life extension programs will be provided as early as possible to extend not just the time everyone has, but also the quality of that time for as long as possible.

Insurance companies will make more money due to a multitude of industry factors that should provide the cost basis for the newly implemented system to thrive for all health care patients and for all providers. The savings from using artificial intelligence in an integrated system with health care will help to regulate the marketplace in a way in which profits should soar for all health insurance companies. There are also many more methodologies of implementation that should return record profits. Due to the upper tiers of right to try being uncapped, pharmaceutical companies should see record profit margins as well.

Since most underwriting divisions in most health care companies have become medical approval divisions, this new system would make possible a drastic reduction in size or even the removal of medical underwriting divisions in each company. Removing almost the entire division would provide massive savings initially. Using artificial intelligence to work in conjunction with each health insurance company's financial goals should permit monetary gain for each company through massive additional savings to net profits that will also come from the rule of large numbers. Eliminating the underwriting division alone for all health care companies should make this program idea viable for all companies.

The rule of large numbers will apply to income for all health insurance companies due to the vast numbers of people being introduced into the private health care marketplace. This inevitable increase is simply due to exponential job growth in many fields of employment. The constant expansion in the number of people gainfully employed means that there will be more individuals buying programs long into the foreseeable future and beyond. Pharmaceutical companies will be able to charge whatever the market will bear for right to try on higher levels of various tiers. This should provide all pharmaceutical companies with record profits immediately and lessen the financial burden that exists under the current model, where wining and dining is necessary for research and development.

With these large numbers, some of the savings will be passed back to the consumer as well. Imagine four gas stations on each corner at the same intersection. Regardless of what is occurring outside of that area to influence pricing, those four gas stations will most likely be competing for the same people to buy their product at that intersection at that moment. The prices will probably be competitive with one another and provide opportunities in many ways for the consumer to save money due to competition among the pricing of the stations. Competition in the health care marketplace with companies crossing state lines is similar. This will create a consumer marketplace where trust is found more readily than under the current model regarding both insurance and pharmaceutical companies. There will be reduced rates for each consumer due to lower monthly costs for group and individual marketplace premiums for each policy, lower costs for patient copays, and smaller deductibles associated with each product choice on every tier. Almost all plans currently in most insurance exchanges were once referred to as and qualified as high-deductible programs, if not all of them at this point in time. Once again, this money will be made back by the companies with the rule of large numbers and tiered program pricing that will be determined by whatever is competitive in the marketplace for each company to decide.

For each health insurance company involved, implementing artificial intelligence in such a manner will save on waste and fraud, require less storage internally, and improve the core communication of all storage applications. Artificial intelligence will also reduce the amount of money necessary for the actual date of procedure cost for each patient and the cost for each company and patient for follow-up care as well. This will be because of improved, highly efficient and exceedingly effective time of immediate care results for patients, which will help to reduce redundant and extraneous visits, and, additionally, because of less time necessary for healing by each patient.

Introducing a tiered system, with multiple different options on each tier, should permit costs to be associated appropriately and all underwriting to be done in a cost-effective manner that permits competition in the marketplace, allowing each company in health care to thrive financially. Oversaturation of the marketplace may provide diluted results; however, competition in the marketplace should serve to regulate consumer costs effectively. The companies that are going to be crossing state lines to provide insurance should be highly regarded and vastly respected for their past performance to ensure the likelihood of improvements in infrastructure, maximizing financial efficiency and guaranteeing quality.

Each state would save money. States will not need to spend as much on individuals in need of state assistance as people come off of state insurance and other state aid programs. This program will save every state an incredible amount of money. Those vast amounts of resources can then be applied to defray the cost of the state educational programs being introduced. That would still leave remaining funds for additional programs to be spent on whatever is necessary for health, survival, and the overall wellbeing of the inhabitants in each state too. Each state would manage its own needs accordingly.

Not everything is equal, even in a stock car race where the entire point is to have everything be the same, hence, stock. There are always different makes of brakes, engines and other parts. These slight variances provide for diverse opportunities at different times, given variant circumstances. Most of life is almost always beyond our ability to have control, and yet we must find ourselves our own path to success on not just any given day, but on every occasion. Instead of running a doomed race that has led to death and decay, with this program, we reinvigorate health care and have the opportunity to be a part of a healthy race.

Stock may not be possible in insurance either, especially state to state with varying cost of living indexes, so be prepared to go with the flow and create all necessary additional adjustments. The requisite accommodation for such programs should be built around the needs of each individual and permit the opportunity for each person to choose what coverage level, cost, and overall plan design specifically meet the needs of each individual and their family's requirements too. Each plan can be described, when put into a package, as a family plan where, in reality, the precise needs of each person in a family are being individualized and structured specifically to help with both prevention and necessary care.

Who owns health care in the state of Colorado? Who owns health care in the state of California? Some state-based insurance companies that were supposed to be run by companies doing business and headquartered within each state under the Affordable Care Act have already been purchased by out of state companies and are now being purchased by companies that are not even incorporated within the United States of America. Sometimes taxes are averted, as health insurance companies are not owned by a company that is owned by a corporation operating its headquarters within the United States of America. It is time for companies to be part of the United States again. If other countries take this plan in the future, their health care companies should eventually be part of their own country, even if assistance is necessary for implementation until that reality may exist.

While some national carriers were initially approved as well, state insurance exchanges were originally started with state specific insurance companies in each state that were to conduct business only in the state in which they were offering insurance products. This was supposedly a mandatory part of the Affordable Care Act. First, these companies were sold to other insurance companies that were participating in the program in order to maintain a structure of insurance integrity identified as part of the organization. Now, some have been sold to out-of-state companies. Since programs are now being designed by out of state insurance companies in most cases already, there should be no problem in permitting insurance companies to do business in states other than those in which they were originally incorporated. This should be done in a capitalistic, competitive business model.

For the environmental learning facilities to work properly and with correct protection, international underwriting insurance companies will play a significant role in securing protection for the financial viability of the project. Companies dealing with hard-to-place coverage and able to use actuaries to determine hard to value projects correctly will flourish, and the creation of these centers will have a tremendous positive impact on their business moving forward. While already available separately in some cases, the concept of health care coverage may eventually be extended through an international tier as well. Travel insurance riders are also necessary, especially for those who need assistance in getting to appointments and other medically related services while abroad.

There also needs to be at least level one health insurance available for people with medical needs, such as acute mental health problems; those seeking temporary housing; and others who are not competent daily to make their own decisions. While limited in scope, this basis will provide annual checkups and emergency care, providing realistic rudimentary requirements. The homeless and the indignant need to be cared for as well. While sensible logistical concerns of life need to always be taken into account, this plan should also reduce dramatically the number of people abusing the health care system.

Insurance requirements should be established for a new line of insurance for residents who do not have the ability to drive, are required not to drive by law due to a restriction, have a mental health condition that prevents their ability to safely operate a vehicle, or are otherwise subject to additional restrictions due to additional equipment management requirements. The criteria for creating a risk assessment and management portfolio for an individual, resident, or participant insurance supplemental passenger policy for vehicular purposes should be established and sent by the undersigned for each policy directly to the insurance company providing coverage. Detailed coverage should be created via rider for any passenger, with the cost dependent upon expected usage and individual necessity. The more frequently a person requires such coverage, the greater the possibility of risk, and hence the more expensive the policy coverage should be. Rates can be determined by each state. Ride share passengers may utilize this concept as a form of new auto insurance, like renters do with some forms of homeowners insurance. Risk assessment models are necessary.

Life insurance programs will be difficult to deal with or, at least, require ingenuity in thought and application as life expectancy increases dramatically for the majority of human beings. Term life insurance options may become temporary necessities to augment current whole life insurance policies. Many, if not most, life insurance policies use a life expectancy of an attained age of one hundred years old for the maturation of the policy. Term life insurance policies are usually able to be purchased by consumers for less money than whole life insurance and are designated for a certain duration. Additionally, term life insurance may be necessary to supplement current whole life insurance policies to reach a new life expectancy age of 121 and then, eventually, much older in the near future. The life insurance industry and all companies doing such business will have to adapt to new regulations and life expectancy expectations on a constant basis for the foreseeable future.

New life insurance products should be examined for different models of existence with longer periods of life experience expected as the norm. This does mean premium adjustments may be necessary. It is possible that some life insurance arrangements and annuity arrangements will have to consider additional coverage opportunities, such as offering additional term life insurance as required riders for existing whole life insurance products in order to help offset any additional issues in the future. Some life insurance products have already started to be based on an attained age necessary for the maturation of the policy of 121 years old; it is possible that this number may very quickly be switched to 150 years of age or even older. Premiums for whole life will still be based upon the actual attained age at the time the policy is purchased by someone. Reevaluation of the marketplace will need to be done on an annual, five-year, and ten-year basis as life expectancy hopefully takes a massive step forward in the immediate future. This will be necessary to ensure proper life insurance policies are available for purchase by the populace so that the industry remains strong. Many different possibilities exist in the future for how to proceed so that consumers and companies remain well protected. This will hopefully allow for all potential needs for all people to be addressed and will suffice as a stabilizing influence on the entire industry of life insurance products available in the future.

This will have an impact on the ability to use life insurance products as investment opportunities. This will also lead to a decrease in the circulation of bad policies being considered and created for use by citizens for possible criminal breaches of behavior, including, but not limited to, fraud and laundering of financial assets. This may include total policy reconsiderations and new recruitment deliberations for eligible citizens to be considered candidates carefully in regard to due process and diligence. Whole life policies, once redesigned for longer life expectancy with fewer financial loopholes, will eventually be the preferable methodology of life insurance again at that juncture for many, if not most, people. New premiums must be created on a scale of life insurance where life expectancy is far greater than the average age is currently estimated to be for most human beings.

While competition in the marketplace should reign supreme for those under 65, Medicare for those over 65 should be universal health care with all coverage provided for everyone, everywhere, every time care is needed. There should be freedom for people to live once they reach a certain stage of life that should not be taken for granted and where mobility is often a difficulty. There is a caveat, though: that much like life insurance, the system will have to be reevaluated in its entirety. The most important provision of this is that the retirement age for Social Security and for Medicare should now be raised to 70 for all people born in the year 2000 or afterwards. In addition, this age should be re-examined every year, as well as every five and ten years, in the context of the average expected life span for human beings as it improves. It is theoretically possible that living to two hundred years old or more could become the expected standard of life expectancy. It is theoretically possible that the average age of life expectancy may grow exponentially versus our current expectations as well. Since this is an expected reality, the need for an overhaul and for continued maintenance towards the concepts of Social Security and Medicare will be a necessity for the foreseeable future. It may be a constant exploration if all works out well.

There are not a great number of lobbyists for the individual when it comes to the health care industry. Moving forward, there should be a prevalence of positive, proactive, preventive patient policies permitting progressive possibilities for meeting all health care needs for all families. Additionally, help will be available to make choices, not just online but in person as well, through insurance brokers in regional and local offices. Complete service will be provided by brokers to help pick anyone up along the way, no matter what or where they may find themselves financially. Brokers will help to facilitate all of the information for each individual and help to create the ideal package year by year for all individuals and families.

A good opportunity for providers to be eligible to offer qualified medical insurance will be obtainable, regardless of whether they currently qualify under the eligibility requirements or not. The time has come for responsible business dealings in all regards to health, from administrators to companies. A service network commitment assurance program will have to be entered into to form the core covenant commitment necessary for each and every company involved to ensure that each participant always actively participates responsibly.

Family is something that should be and is revered as a cornerstone of any and all societies. Family planning is essential when it comes to creating new relationships with health care providers, health care institutions, and health care practitioners, including specialists, with health care infrastructure that provides services related to individual illnesses. This will include family plans from insurance providers that provide services related to the individual needs of everyone in each family. Services will be provided differently under diverse types of plans and on numerous types of available tiers. Some programs will include a la carte options instead of traditional programs, whereas in other instances, coverage will still be available through more traditional programs that have been implemented previously, with various additional riders available.

Ideally, in the future, to assist families, all disabled children will be awarded at least the third tier of health insurance coverage automatically and each disabled child will receive whatever coverage is necessary for their health and well-being for life. This brings up the innate concept that all children should be awarded health insurance coverage automatically with whatever tier and program are necessitated for their health too. This coverage will expire at the age of eighteen unless a person is permanently disabled due to a preexisting condition that necessitates future care. Realistically, though, this idea for how to provide health insurance for all children will have to wait. While possible for disabled children immediately, if this portion of the system were implemented for all children now, it may collapse the entire health care system as it is currently structured. While the rest of this system is achievable and realistic here and now, this change is not. Unfortunately, it is currently not feasible to achieve complete oversight and overhaul of the health care system's insurance marketplace to realize even more for all children without overwhelming the system with undue financial risk, burden and pressure. The rest of this program works immediately with any and all other considerations, though. Hopefully, with abundant resources, a proper balance between financial necessity and moral integrity can be better balanced soon for all people.

When it comes to the concept of health, success should be measured by patient results and satisfaction. Each family and person needs to be able to choose what health insurance coverage works best for that person and their family in tiered concierge a la carte insurance programs. These are inventive program initiatives that encourage each family to design their own health coverage that works for each and all individuals in the family. This will permit the ability for the collective family unit to know that every person in that household is covered correctly. This should provide for increased consumer satisfaction and comfort so that each member of the family will be confident that they will get the care necessary if needed.

Individualized, streamlined care for all patients starts with being able to pick the right insurance program that works for that person and, separately, the right pharmaceutical options that are necessary for each individual and fit his or her life accordingly. Having access to the care each person needs on a cost-effective basis is a necessity for all people. This is where providing health insurance in a new manner provides the opportunity for innovative magic that binds us all together in appreciation of things we share in a real way, with good service being of high importance in all phases of the health care and insurance industries. The goal is for every person to be able to receive good care when expected, and realizing that goal means good care is obtained by every single person when needed. This plan will initiate smart modernizations in the entire health care industry. Families want to live a happy, healthy, heartfelt life together for as many years as possible. It is time to have the insurance industry provide a path for all families and individuals to be healthy.

CHAPTER 7

EDUCATION – CHANGES IN APPROACHES TO LEARNING

Our health care system is irrevocably broken, insufficient, and dangerous. The purpose of the statement initially sought to provide a foundation for health for all children and families. In discovering what is necessary to remedy the system, certain undeniable realities emerged: fixing the foundation of health care requires a multitude of other considerations to be addressed simultaneously. The purpose of providing health for all shall always be what this statement was created for, will stand for, and will forever be about. Also, putting the concept into action with care and consideration is of vital importance. Both the implementation and the realization of this new system of health care must be done with love. This is especially true and necessary when compared to today's environment and experience for most children, young people, and all others. In that vein, education reform is the first necessary alteration in creating a healthier society.

School needs to be a comfortable environment for all students and all children to feel relaxed, empathetic, respectful, knowledgeable, appreciated, and able to feel that someone cares about them. It is vitally important that children experience life with love being shown consistently so that they may grow to have kindness, knowledge, compassion, and love in all manners of life. With the foundation of a new educational format of learning established, all children will have the opportunity to experience the freedom to soar together to heighten their prospects of a new tomorrow that we cannot even imagine today.

Let us make sure that every single opportunity for orphaned children matches in every single way the opportunity given to children who may have ample prospects. It is important that all children feel that they have every single chance possible, regardless of any other circumstance. Achieving this concept is the realization necessary for equality of opportunity and provides the basis for equality to be realized in action for the rest of time.

All children should have faith and confidence that they will win the championship when they are called upon to deliver for themselves and for all of society, and that when that time comes and they are called upon, each and every one of those children will know in their heart, essence, soul, and in every fiber of their being that they are prepared and ready to hit the game winning grand slam, sink the putt that counts, score the game winning goal, complete the race, cross the goal line for the touchdown to win the game in overtime, make the game winning shot, and even dunk it with authority. We must teach our children to just be the best possible people that they can be every single day with faith that their lives matter and that together they will win every championship possible for the rest of time.

The education programs of tomorrow will far exceed those of today, with total customization for comfort for all learners, adapted to all learning thought patterns, learning methods, and all styles of learning for all students. Adapting to learning abilities and time schedules for certification achievements for all learning thought participants of any age who are interested should also provide an atmosphere where education is fun and exciting, and motivation may increase dramatically. This will permit test scores to ascend and each student to maximize his or her learning opportunities to the utmost of his or her potential.

Just because a year went by does not mean everyone picked up the information requisite to have truly understood and mastered the annual curriculum of that school or calendar year. We all have different learning methods and styles for processing and retaining information. Flowers do not all bloom at once; in fact, flowers bloom at different times of the year, which is very much like children blooming in their education at different times in their lives. This is true for almost all of us as we weave through life; we all evolve and, hopefully, eventually in a healthy manner, become our best friends to ourselves on our own individual path and time schedule in life, and that cannot be forgotten or taken for granted. Streamlined and individualized educational training activities would be a wonderful addition to primary education for every student.

Our children are being forced to navigate through a hate filled, narcissistic, selfish jungle of a journey. With no real opportunity to succeed, they will eventually be forced to devour one another. They live in a world of social media predators where social media has become a predator itself in how our children are spending their time and in the things that preoccupy their minds that may not be healthy.

Since the Comstock Act of 1873, there have been restrictions on the distribution of obscene material. So, what happened with the internet? Why are our children now subject to offensive material all the time? Trouble used to be that thing found outside of the home; now it finds its way inside every day.

We need to end violence in our schools now and forever. No child should ever have to fear going to school due to the possibility of tragedies that have plagued the youth of our country far too often over the past couple of decades. The once unheard of has become entirely too commonplace. Artificial intelligence will help to provide deterrents to having such incidents occur in the future. AI will provide instant feedback as to which children are truly at risk rather than relying on the personal interpretations that have been proven incorrect so often. Rather than depending on guesses, artificial intelligence will provide advance notice of possible concerns when appropriate. Instead of concern over what was previously unforeseeable, this should permit all parents to focus on making their children successful while feeling that their children are in a safe environment during class. The most important part of these advances will be that every child should be able to worry more about recess than about another atrocity occurring.

The number one reason why having time is important is shown by the current lack of proper parenting, as parents are not spending time with their children. This is not an attack; it could be simply that the parent or parents are decimated after a long workday and do not have any energy left; however, even in the most reasonable of circumstances, such as this example, it is the children who are left being damaged by an inability to spend the time necessary for proper guidance. Mostly, it leaves a very cold world where even the most loved children feel alone and sad.

Even when families get together and sit at the dinner table these days, it is a far cry from the days of yore when families ate almost every meal together. Nowadays, one person may be watching television while one other person is on their computer, and another person is on a tablet while still another is on their phone. Sharing our days and asking each other about how the other person's day was is important for many reasons. It has become a lost, exceptionally important concept, and its demise has shattered the dreams, homes, and lives of people. It is time to revive the concept of active listening, especially with our family.

Parents' spending time with their children, whether it be going outside to play, going to sporting activities or to outside recreational fun places, museums, places of science, habitat exploration, or even just talking during dinner, has profound effects on what a child learns and the inspiration those thoughts create. Parents should make children look stuff up for themselves and then make sure they understand the information by making sure the children use the information in a sentence relevant to demonstrating their understanding. A very good methodology to make sure someone has learned something is the concept of watch one, do one, then teach one on any given subject matter to see how well an individual understands and has truly mastered something, too.

Children sometimes seemingly even learn by osmosis, and simply being around culture, knowledge, and understanding can sometimes provoke enough stimulus of thought that the child at hand can master concepts seemingly beyond their years and even develop new thoughts that are far beyond the original comprehension of the material at hand. Being immersed in a world of daydreams can inspire thought patterns that revolutionize the world and bring new understandings never before dreamed of by anyone previously. This evolutionary pattern of thought has often shaped the world.

According to philosophy and psychology literature, researchers question whether knowledge quality leads to an increased quality of understanding through knowledge development rather than knowledge acquisition. In other words, gymnastics and recreational activities may teach functional reasoning at a much higher level than traditional educational methods within the classroom setting. It is important to learn more about individual learning methods and proper environments for permitting functional activities in the classroom to reinforce knowledge acquisition through the usage of knowledge development.

Education is a vital necessity. It should be fun to learn, too. Music, art, and gym are where you apply the sciences in school. These classes need to be prioritized again. Just like athletic events, there need to be scholastic events with schools matching knowledge and wits against each other, including qualifying for playoffs and taking home trophies for being tough enough to be smart enough to be champions.

Early childhood developmental courses will be occasionally available in specific situations for those with high aptitude and special learning capabilities on an appropriately healthy, expedited learning curve, without forgetting that they, too, still need to be kids, though. We are all children at heart. Maintaining that heart is just as important as proper education.

There should be an emphasis on technology and cutting-edge equipment that need to be provided in all possible classrooms so that hands-on learning may be done by all students. Visualizing a concept by seeing it in action can spark imagination vividly. There should also be logistics training in a variety of different trades and activities, from cooking to sewing to budget management. Learning how to cook, clean, and be financially responsible together means civilization may be able to truly see the next generation, and all future generations, be a team going forward, united forever and ever with understanding and compassion.

Enrollment opportunities should not be limited in any possible field of endeavor, nor should any path of educational pursuit be restricted. All programs will be available for blind individuals and deaf persons, as well as for those with any other difficulty that must be overcome in order to have educational opportunities facilitated. Enrollment opportunities for all should happen in a wide variety of fields, as previously discussed. In regard to the environmental learning centers, there will also be additional programs for consideration as time permits, including, but not limited to, agrarian and other health-related fields. Neuroinclusivity is a necessity of learning.

Future Farmers of America (FFA) already has many agrarian courses and training available across a wide spectrum of knowledge and activities in relation to farming and agriculture. It is innate in reality that these endeavors of our past will always be useful, as they present necessary survival skills that are still useful today and will always be useful in our future as well. This leads to the inescapable conclusion that agricultural knowledge and studies are inherently part of health and should be included in the undergraduate study programs available. A Community Supported Agriculture (CSA) week of free farming lessons may be integrated as part of a summer study course that allows children, adolescents, high school, and college students to learn about the importance of agriculture. 4-H may be able to offer agriculture and hands-on veterinary preparation activities, thus helping all children with his or her head, heart, hands, and health in the future. Local garden clubs may assist with recreational opportunities for understanding flora growth. These courses may also provide a school opportunity for learning self-sufficiency, even for those with different pursuits.

Artificial intelligence may also permit studies into previously seemingly unrelated fields that may possibly create entirely new fields of study, disciplines, and remedies moving forward. Insects and their properties are such an example. This will take time to prove; however, it is conceivable that there are some correlating factors that would provide entirely new ideas on how to proceed with health care in the medical industry for humans.

Bed bugs have a natural coagulant and are attracted to carbon dioxide, which may help as a warning system and for understanding carbon issues affecting health. Bed bugs and tardigrades, a form of microscopic cockroaches, seemingly produce their own natural antiseptic. Ants have been around for fifty million years and are able to perform their own waste removal of unnecessary leafing and other environmental hazards through antibacterial secretions of their own. It is possible that this may help the study of disinfectants. Studies may indicate how to create sterile environments that are easier to keep antiseptic and provide opportunities for a multitude of applications in various fields.

From aardvarks to zebras, animals have feelings too. Just as horses are regal animals, we all are. Whether we are mustangs, stallions, or even more of a trotter, it is up to us to decide how we wish to run the race ahead for ourselves. All animals need us to supply a healthier planet Earth moving forward. For us to soar with the falcons and the eagles, we must make sure all animals know that we are their friends and are concerned about their health, habitats, and environments. After all, the world that we provide for the animals is the one we shall be providing for ourselves, our children and the future, too.

Wild turkeys are highly intelligent, family oriented and caring animals that were so highly regarded by Benjamin Franklin that he recommended that turkeys be the official bird of the United States of America before the country finally settled on the bald eagle as its official bird symbol of the country. Horses are regarded as animals who are highly intelligent and have real connections with the people who ride them and take care of them. Dogs, cats, and other animals are family members.

Animals are faithful companions. Perfect symmetry is found in a symbiotic relationship between humans, animals, and Earth, and now artificial intelligence, which will help. Balance must be achieved for the long-term health of all involved. The animals' territories and the whole environment of Earth that can be positively maintained should be taken care of as a precious habitat for existence for all people, creations, and animals. Every geographic location should be protected and provided for in a healthy manner for it to always survive, too. The environmental learning centers, and the educational opportunities they will provide, will be beneficial to all life forms. Courses in environmental research, agrarian training and veterinary studies will be available to all students at these institutions.

Veterinary surgical centers and hospitals should be available at the same location so that care and aftercare for animal surgeries can allow for less interference and a reduced need to travel to multiple places for care. A veterinary surgery and animal hospital in one place will facilitate care in case of an emergency. In addition, there will be an animal ambulance service with veterinarians who can travel to make house calls. The ability to perform surgeries on animals should be greatly enhanced by communication advances. Almost all of these advances in health care for human beings are also available for animals and make it possible for an animal to be part of a life extension program moving forward, too. All necessary amendments that need to be made should be completed, as all pets are family and should be protected as such with insurance and with up-to-date health care facilities. There will be access to affordable health care and health care insurance for all animals and pets. Expect a tiger to cost more than a house cat, though.

Impending improvements in the audio and video capabilities of artificial intelligence will lead to the possibility of animal transmission being translated into various languages. A veterinarian will have language training and will utilize a language translation system deemed appropriate for usage when dealing with animals for treatment. Animal translation will be included as part of a large, encompassing approach to creating a health care facility for veterinary services that provides full-service interventions, procedures, education, and management facilities, along with the ability to support all veterinary applications for all animals. Just as education is evolving for doctors and nurses, veterinary studies are also advancing rapidly as well.

There should be access to safe, reasonable, appropriate housing for all animals that need temporary boarding and at an affordable rate. Healthy housing facilities will be developed that are better and safer than current kennel standards with more room for pets to roam free. Part of the advancement of educational programs for children will include state of the art facilities where it is possible to incorporate some of the housing concepts into an educational format where children are able to spend time hands-on with different animals.

Every child will have opportunities that are real and attainable. No more will there be limitations due to societal ills. It is time to remedy our school and education system once and for all, no matter what. Youth services must be dramatically improved during the implementation process immediately. The money being saved from a reduction of people requiring government aid should permit new programs to help educate children. If necessary, family shelters ought to be available for temporary short-term stay requirements, with the child's education being of paramount importance as to why and where the aid is distributed. Once instituted, all students will have access as well.

Orphans will not be left behind anymore, as they will share the same opportunities as every other person with the newly reformed educational opportunities of being able to pursue a degree as a doctor, nurse, farmer, or veterinarian regardless of any other circumstance. Orphans frequently experience intense feelings of abandonment, loneliness, grief, anxiety, identity issues, feelings of unworthiness, and depression. Being left alone may lead to a loss of security and trust issues, which can lead to difficulties in forming future attachments to other people. With the revamping of local schoolhouses, all deprived children and orphans will be loved with the same food and education programs available to all other children.

The autism spectrum of learning applies to all of us, as there is a spectrum for all of us in many different stations and situations in life, especially in how we learn and process information. How do we really know what it feels like to go through the same thing as someone else? We make assumptions that we understand and are being compassionate in our endeavors; however, we truly cannot walk in someone else's shoes or literally see through their eyes. We all learn differently and at diverse rates from one another.

To achieve a truly erudite society, the theory of autism brilliance needs to be investigated further. Sometimes, those thought initially to be limited in possibilities due to their autism become brilliant contributors in a variety of different fields with thought patterns that have not been contemplated previously. In fact, often, overcoming the learning difficulties that feel overwhelming today leads to a strength of character and fortitude of one's soul that seemingly creates superpowers that are necessary to create the evolution that empowers all of us and lead to educational advancements for all people tomorrow. Those that appear to be gallivanting around today may transform into our charismatic, compassionate, brilliant leaders of tomorrow.

Education will have more information influencing cure and innovation. Information influences the delivery of a system, and this new culture of education will provide improved results and allow for expedited evolution of souls, bodies and minds. That is a far better value for the money than what is currently spent on educational resources and will be forever as from now on value will be determined by what is best for the student population.

Educating the masses should help all people go as far as each person's ambition permits, satiate any of the innate desires for achievement that vary for each of us, while also making a huge difference in our individual hearthstones. This is significant because it lays a point of foundation for what types of religion, government, and other types of pursuits we happen to formulate a proclivity and proclamation for. Most of the difficulty of creating this change is just part of the process and eventually leads to increased happiness, incredible wealth, and fulfillment, with children and young people always being a part of our lives moving forward.

Scruples permit opportunities to review information and determine the authenticity and validity of application. They may also provide opportunities for false information to be provided, and this requirement applies to all information transmitted as it relates to all honest communication. Sometimes going forward with our initial instinctive institutional instructions that we feel inherently during the inception of our thought patterns provides the best course of action and opportunities for advancement to achieve a correct diagnosis. In other words, let us not second guess our way out of being right to begin with when going with our gut will lead us to the correct answer to begin with; let not our fear overcome us.

Simply put, the doctor does not go home with the patient, and the patient does not necessarily need to know exactly everything the doctor does to appreciate the doctor, even if the patient pontificates as such sometimes later. It is always dangerous to assume that, just because someone articulates something correctly, the patient or the people involved heard the message being expressed. It does not matter what is said; what matters is what is heard and understood. People have different forms of communication. Sometimes words or expressions can have different meanings for different people. Communication is not solely about being heard; it is about understanding and conversational considerations. Usually, this means active listening is important to learn how to convey a message in a way that the receiver comprehends the message being sent so as to not lead to an empty note.

There is a very difficult balance to reach in the modern era of education, and while reforms are necessary, there are some very difficult conversations that need to be had as to the realities of life. Covering for a lack of care at home for some students really does elevate the teacher into the role as the most important positive influence in some children's lives. This is balanced by those parents who are actively engaged in the lives of their children and have no control over the curriculum that could be a cause for consternation. Consideration of appropriateness is sometimes seemingly totally disregarded, which tends to provide an atmosphere of exacerbation with extracurriculars instead of education in the essentials.

There is truth in that with some teacher dominated opinions on curriculum and teaching methodologies, there are specific times when certain students are being indoctrinated rather than educated. The difference is that indoctrination is teaching somebody what to think, while education is teaching an individual how to think for themselves. This can limit critical reasoning skills, and those skills are sometimes necessary for survival, especially with life and death decisions that are often instantaneous and unforeseen in life. The better someone is taught to think for themselves, the better prepared that person will be when life dictates situations that may have dire consequences.

Teaching is creating the ability to allow someone to think for themselves. Understand that teaching someone what to think is important for certain people, rather than causing them to harm themselves unnecessarily; however, otherwise, doing so leads to indoctrination and limits the ability of those people to have the best possible development for psychological adaptation in certain highly structured or stressful environments, which are inevitable for all of us in our daily lives, including in accordance with other environmental factors. The mere introduction of indoctrination can lead to a person having a much more difficult time than they need to in some situations in life versus when that same person is provided with the ability to think for themselves in all circumstances with critical reasoning skills that have been developed. It can even lead to a lack of confidence, loss of interest in various activities, and becoming dependent on others just to survive on a daily basis for the rest of their lives.

Learning is not about parroting information back to the teacher and getting good grades for doing so. Learning is about discovering the abilities necessary to think for oneself and be able to integrate successfully into a multitude of different situations and environments over the course of a lifetime. Learning multiple languages, mathematical bases, and varying cultures permits more than just knowing that the way to perform the conversion from Celsius to Fahrenheit is to take the Celsius number, multiply by 9, divide by 5, and add 32: $(X°C \times 9/5) + 32$. Learning as much as possible to be able to think for oneself provides the basis for any person to be able to overcome obstacles that ostensibly always occur in life.

Teaching someone how to fish is at least figuratively important and an awesome thing to do, even if you are a crappy fisherman, because the next generation may be far better at fishing. It is possible that the next generation may learn or even invent new ways of doing things far better than was known to be possible beforehand. Also, knowing how to fish is even more important if you need to eat and do not control access to the fish.

Teachers, administrators, and staff, including psychologists, will be required to attend yearly educational meetings and also must meet proper supervision standards set forth by each school, school system, and state and federal guidelines. Education for professionals from kindergarten through all education levels shall be maintained and measured appropriately so that opportunities are representative of performance and education provided in a result-based fashion of competence demonstrated by the student population. This will be done by simply giving the same test at the end of the school year that was given on the first day of class. These tests will be varied depending on factors such as previously demonstrated ability and will match the age-appropriate goals for developing students while encouraging expansion.

To ensure that teachers are of the highest quality and character, there will be qualifications for certain characteristics established under the jurisdiction of each state's board of education and the federal government. This will include a questionnaire evaluation exercise that will be undertaken under the jurisdiction in charge of that geographical area. The subsequent assessment administered will be presented along with appropriate amendments available across the jurisdiction to make sure standards are upheld in order to qualify and afterwards, too.

There will be training qualifications for all participants. In order to find qualified, knowledgeable graduate students who may be able to assist as teachers' aides for teachers, there will be a questionnaire evaluation exercise undertaken every year under the jurisdiction of the board of education. Resulting assessment information will determine what needs to be administered along the way for improvements to constantly be made by all members of the school system, so the education of every child is top notch in every way.

It is imperative to finally answer the question of what quality education needs. This means that it is necessary to improve understanding and knowledge of management of education through constant assessment. The questions are hard enough to quantify, such as what is necessary for quality improvement; however, questions not asked can quickly lead to a regression of educational foundation and understanding. This same concept of education exploration enhancement questions will be true in all fields of enterprise evolving eventually. Expanding educational expertise will facilitate our interactions with additional learners from other professions. Our life experiences will be utilized to optimize education for all students moving forward. Providing integrated learning throughout the university structure, including performance evaluation and suggestions for improvement, will provide exponential opportunities for experiential learning across the entire spectrum of university preparation choices. Also, it will create entirely new possibilities for varying structures of curriculum that should become more prevalent, accepted, and necessary over time.

Reopening old schools that are available as academic environments of safety is needed right now and will require volunteer staffing in addition to finding funds for a large-scale number of new teachers. Volunteerism is a necessity to keep neighborhoods and communities clean and safe for all. The money for these new teaching jobs will be found in the forecast model and will be possible from the number of people coming off of state aid and federal aid programs. In the interim, credits from post-graduate institutions for higher education will help, as they may provide teaching opportunities in elementary educational settings for current students in various fields. Everyone and anyone who contributes to the success of this venture will be a paragon of virtue, eliciting positivity together.

Education in smaller schools, such as the small school-houses of yesterday, would help to provide a more independent, inclusive educational experience and environment for all students. This would permit the proper ability to make sure that every student has the opportunity to experience education evolution, where time is taken at the appropriate pace and the necessary individual methodology is applied to each student.

Also, smaller educational centers for learning, being more localized, will serve to reduce carbon emissions. This will be accomplished simply by reducing the amount of carbon, a goal that is expected to be achieved by reducing the amount of carbon actually created and by increasing the amount of school settings and buildings that can be established while reducing, maybe also eliminating in some areas, the number of school buses that would previously have needed to be used for transporting students. Simply put, these programs will help to severely reduce carbon emissions, with fewer buses being utilized, as students will be closer to home. Also, the money given for school buses annually in each state's budget could be used for providing additional programs, books, educational materials, and field trip opportunities for the students, while still providing abundant savings for each state.

Neighborhood education systems would reduce the number of buses and hence reduce the number of children needing to ride buses to get a proper education. Doing so would result in dramatically lower carbon emissions and drastically reduce air pollution in vulnerable communities while simultaneously reducing the carbon footprint and environmental concerns of impoverished communities. Also, this idea would result in fewer children waiting to catch the bus in adverse weather, which often leads to a communal illness that requires time to run through the entire education system. In fact, local neighborhood school settings should permit more children everywhere the ability to walk to school and back home, which is exponentially healthier for the children themselves. As a byproduct, this may also help to reduce childhood obesity rates in the United States. We need to foster an effective environment of positivity and health for all. There is never a need to ever adversely affect a student's health, mind, opportunities, or wellbeing.

Kids are expensive, especially for single moms and dads; the schoolhouse idea helps to save money and time. It would also help to extend hours at the schoolhouses as necessary for such situations to meet the needs of those parents whose work schedules are not conducive to normal practices, especially the ones established currently. Regionalism, defined as neighborhood settings, can help single moms and dads and all parents with time as well as ease and comfort. Providing extended-hour opportunities for parents who work differently than what is normally available will allow for healthier environments.

Even with help programs like Care for Kids, education is expensive and hard to afford; this is especially true for single parent households. Other new education help programs are also needed, as raising a child is becoming more expensive. While these educational centers are becoming more effective in helping to raise children and while families are becoming more educated in how to help their children, the cost of raising children has become cost-prohibitive for some. Small schoolhouse settings qualify for education money allowances granted by the federal government, reducing all associated costs at the state level as well.

Libraries may make good use of space for neighborhood school services. Oftentimes, there can be free stuff for students with a library card, such as when students go online to https://hoopla.com. Additionally, a library of things is not just information; however, it contains actual things that are available and useful for necessary activities. These include various household tools and materials available temporarily for anyone to borrow as necessary.

Wallingford, Connecticut's collaborative library has cutting edge learning items and is a fine example of providing a modern, new age learning environment where the students will be engaged and enthralled by the advancements of today while discovering the possibilities of tomorrow. This concept of hands-on learning being more readily available provides advantages in more areas, helping to propel all of society into a new evolutionary plan for success. These libraries are an investment in any local area's citizenry and milieu.

In the United States of America, there should be a concentration of effort to preserve antiquity by providing protection for history forgotten by employing local dedicated preservation of farmlands and caution for empty spaces of importance. The agricultural history around a place like the University of Connecticut should provide a brilliant opportunity for land conservancy. Precedents for such endeavors have been achieved previously, such as the Acropolis preservation in Greece. The historical safeguarding of land, especially significant historical buildings and areas, is a necessity to preserve the cultural heritage, historic context, textures, and realities of a given time. Protection of churches, fields, and other buildings of historical significance will help us to understand the past from long ago well into the future. There needs to be conservation of artifacts in towns, as some relics are being absolutely abandoned and absorbed into the new street developments, shopping, and industrial areas in towns. Unfortunately, these artifacts are then lost forever because of the construction, and then these pieces of history are simply forgotten about.

Antiques and collectibles of importance should be preserved as well. The collection may be anything from medallions from a specific era to bowls from certain dynasties. From Remington statues to even buildings such as St. Peter's Basilica in Vatican City, preservation helps us to remain tethered to the truth. It is vital to preserve with integrity, honor, and reverence, especially since establishing legacy is important. While the days of the Yankee peddler are long since gone, the wares provided may still be worth maintaining for posterity. Old antique cars would be a wonderful idea for science conservation. People who do not know the past are often doomed to repeat it. Preservation promotes peace.

The costs associated with becoming a student have become prohibitive for most individuals, especially the costs associated with becoming a student at a post-secondary education university for instructive purposes such as medical school. Law enforcement, law education, and financial educational career opportunities sometimes take years after schooling is completed for a return on investment to be seen by the student. These careers often require internships even after postgraduate education is completed. The scope of this for any student enrolled in university programs may mean that they will never get out of financial debt when what they are going to school for is to provide themselves with the opportunity to be free to have their own pursuit of happiness. There is an unfortunate irony in the process of pursuing higher education only to be met with living in a parent's basement after successfully completing that education for far too many people right now.

The cost for people wanting to become doctors, especially surgical physicians, is increasing, and economic factors now play a major role in determining who can pursue becoming a doctor as a career path. Becoming a doctor may mean many more years of experience and education after graduating from postgraduate university studies; sometimes it requires three to eight additional years of education for specific training and accreditation. Due to financial constraints, we have made it almost impossible for our best and our brightest to even be able to become surgical doctors or general physicians. This has also led to a situation where there are thousands of doctors who are educated; however, these individuals may not be as altruistic as one may believe. In fact, currently, many patients feel that their doctors have a high degree of narcissism and do not always exhibit the most appropriate or acceptable bedside management skills.

Implementing the new educational format of opportunities discussed should be relatively easy in certain states. Some states are already offering the basis of this program with their state community college courses being offered for free as of now at all community colleges that are funded by the state. All other state funded assistance programs being provided by the state are already available at these locations. In addition, all federal government subsidies are already available at these institutions of higher learning. The associated costs for people attending, state governments, and the federal government should be more than acceptable on all financial levels immediately. In reality, the associated costs are already expected and allocated for by most students, state governments, and the federal government for the first two years of the education process. All additional future federal government assistance will provide easier access to all in-person classes and online learning mechanisms as well as assist with all other associated required costs, such as housing and food.

There will have to be at least a certain amount of financial reorganization within the university fund allocation process within the academic year moving forward for the subsequent milestones discussed previously to be achieved. There are significant challenges that will need to be addressed, such as securing qualified teachers, administrators, technicians, researchers and volunteers. The proper structuring of financial resources in advance of the new program initiative should lend itself to a prosperous long-term financial dividend after the initial investment is made for all secondary institutions of learning.

Another example of where institutions of higher education do not have access to the resources needed to meet the requirements that will soon be established as base enrollment guidelines necessary under the strategies proposed will be the amount of available space for dormitories. This should be planned for in advance and funds should be invested by the board of trustees for a major return on investment after implementation of the education and training necessary to accomplish quality standards within the university.

These recommendations for reorganization are going to be discussed with the leadership committee of each individual university. A proper balance between funding and administrative support should be discussed immediately, thought through diligently, and then concluded quickly so that implementation of the education program can be initiated as soon as possible. Discussions about budgets will continue, as future needs should be met as demonstrated necessary during the implementation of the education program for long-term viability and success.

Increasing the possibility of affording university studies may also help adoption rates, as prospective parents may feel more capable of providing a secure, safe community and a comfortable environment, which may enhance the viability of adoption abilities. It is possible that organizations such as the Dave Thomas Foundation will be part of this process, as these opportunities will go to all children now. Tax breaks for adopting parents will make it easier for adoption rates and educational rates to increase.

There will be no more teenage wasteland due to student debt. If the average student takes on $200000 in student loan debt, the odds are that the student who accumulates such debt while in school will have a very difficult time paying off that debt during the course of their lifetime, if they are ever able to pay off the debt at all. If the amount of debt continues to compound with interest over the years, and without a guarantee of employment, it is possible that higher education will come to be looked at with a growing distaste in favor of vocational school employment preparation. Some students suffering from such debt obligations have already started to move outside of the United States to avoid defaulting.

The average annual tuition cost has grown to be astronomical and unaffordable for most people. The University of California at Berkeley has an in state tuition cost of $46000 per year for 2025 and an out of state tuition cost of $78,500 per year, while it is $88300 per year to attend Harvard and

$92333 per year to attend Stanford; and while the University of Connecticut is a great state institution, it is hard to believe that it is currently $36000 per year for in state students to attend UConn and $58500 for out of state students. A private school like Skidmore College in Saratoga Springs, New York, costs around $89300 per year to attend. All of these costs are for the undergraduate departments of education and show the tremendous difficulty that most students will have in attempting to pay off their student loan debt.

For what universities are asking for tuition costs in modern times, room and board should be included for all students and families. Sports and donations always provide more opportunities for university students to diversify their amenities and living conditions, especially at major state funded institutions. There should be access to safe, affordable housing for all students and their families.

Profiles seem to mean more than reality to the point that there is no interview as part of the process for most people when they are applying for some university studies in the modern world. There is currently around a 1% acceptance rate for international students at Stanford University and less than 5% at Harvard within the context of qualifications at those institutions of higher learning. Skidmore, for instance, has a 38% acceptance rate for international students.

In the new program, any people living within a territory that the United States is responsible for, such as Puerto Rico or Samoa, will also be immediately eligible for all educational benefits. This will include access to the collection of courses essential for any duration of time that is necessary to complete all prerequisites to be eligible for the college courses. The inclusion of people from these environments should also promote growth for possible hospital infrastructures to be created in the future. This should promote prosperous peace.

There is something to be said for the fact that patience is a virtue. For all people, taking a year or two after high school to dedicate themselves to an outside endeavor to aid the community as a whole before entering college or university may permit time for self-knowledge. This time may provide an opportunity to grow as a person and for maturation to present a path to what a person truly wants to study in college. Everyone is different, and so is what we want to study. Taking the time necessary to develop may also make the expenditure for university studies more worthwhile for the individual as well, as a directed focus on what a person wants to achieve in life may have become more readily apparent.

This process may also provide a citizenship path for families currently dealing with deportation so that the young students who have already been living in the United States of America have a pathway to earn the right to call the USA their permanent home. Through four years of active service in the military or volunteering at the environmental learning centers or other accredited institutions that become integrated into positive success for all, a path will be provided so that no one may ever question the validity of the responsibility accepted by the individual in such a situation. Hence, this should provide a way to make a positive out of a perceived negative for every child and create peace instead of despair.

Viva la Libertad forever, especially when it comes to all children being able to have quality educational opportunities. Let the bagpipes be heard far and wide, for we shall discover buried treasures and aspire for all of our children to live as kings and queens and as masters of their own domain and be the unimpeded creators of each of their own destinies. We and all future generations will be custom crafted carpentry crusaders with an everlasting angelic light enlightening with a soft, delicate, kind, gentle touch in a premier down-to-earth bonded union, holding on until we build a whole new legacy that is only always one stone away at a time.

Each of us has our own journey. We also all have a shared journey together as well. Information and knowledge are really important, as they are the basic tenets of real power and must be used properly so they may be a positive force driving us forward into all unknowns. Getting in sync takes time and is hard; however, the long history of evolution reminds us it is also what makes us ready to climb the long hill ahead and find success at the apex of existence together in every way.

Let us discover synergy together using the good old classroom idea of communication while demonstrating classification achieved appropriately so as not to inhibit education while promoting a classic version of information transfer that permits the deluxe capabilities of true achievement. Be the person that helps to fuel the collaboration of technology and humanity into a system that prioritizes the health, education, and future of all our children forever and ever.

What is on tap is us creating harmony by finding and striking the right chords together in united love. We all shall have detailed creations available for our own pursuits that allow us to see each of us be as smart as possible. Our ingenuity will have us dancing on air with the viability to thrive beyond any limits, replace the carousel of life with rocket starships of new possibilities, and do so with the integrity of the original intent of the Hippocratic oath. We will do everything as individuals in an integrated reality of a collective of one for eternity.

CHAPTER 8

ENVIRONMENTAL LEARNING CENTERS

There is an equation that usually leads to good luck; it is when preparation meets opportunity. When this occurs, good luck is generally demonstrated in any pursuit of life. The creation of these environmental learning centers will create special opportunities for everyone. Due to the fact that these centers will be operating in diverse locations throughout the world, there will inevitably be various opportunities for employment and careers in fields never thought of before.

Environmental learning centers will be placed by the United States of America, investors, and other countries that choose to participate in some of the most inhospitable and volatile places on Earth. Each will be there with the purpose of understanding our planet and how to keep Earth healthy, with the goal of instituting plans that work to maintain the health of our world in a highly efficient manner moving forward. These will include volcanic, oceanic, desert, jungle, swamp, farmland, mountain, and riverside environmental learning centers. All centers will be necessary for examining and understanding the potential impacts of various environmental conditions, identifying possible remedies for cleaning and treatment of dangerous ecological circumstances, and repairing the deadly damage already done to the Earth.

Some of these locations will be in severely harsh environments and will require such things as evacuation personnel. All participants would benefit if those employed for evacuation purposes had prior training, especially military preparation, even special operations training, that permits the bravest, fiercest, and most reliable to flourish. Special forces will be helpful, especially for the unforeseen. Everything will be up to 11A standards and more, from infantry to computers, bolts, amplifiers and energy relays. Handicapped people who are wheelchair bound and all other qualified applicants will have excellent career opportunities as drone operators, especially with prior military training. Hopefully, those who served with distinction and are not physically capable of being on active duty find that they have found a new way to serve with honor, valor and commitment.

In the longer term, job opportunities will be plentiful, with everything from crossing guards to special openings required for securing the safety of the inhabitants of these structures. These environmental learning centers will have to be improved considerably after initial implementation and will be assessed constructively in a manner consistent with the needs of the people living in those structures. Every space must have proper acoustic designs. Artificial intelligence will help to design the noise regulation from classrooms to music rooms to living quarters. From the inception of creation at each center, the management of greenhouse gas emissions and all other necessities of building the environmental learning centers, as well as amenities that will eventually be part of the structures, such as restaurants, schools, normal daily business functions, and all manner of business, should be accounted for initially, as there will eventually be merchants and inhabitants of all sorts.

Sprinklers for fire protection, with advances in sprinkler systems for other purposes such as vegetative growth and agrarian uses, will be another area of advancement that will be necessary for these centers to operate safely and with proper efficiency. Firefighting foam and fans will be other parts of necessary implementations for fire prevention.

There will have to be ingenuity applied to various possible scenarios in advance that are unusual to modern building structures. As such, advancements in the fields of architectural design, safety, artificial intelligence, engineering, and other fields of endeavor may dictate how and when to operate these individual environmental learning centers successfully and will have to be looked upon immediately. Those possible fields that need to be used to be prepared for various situations of necessity may even dictate how, and even where, to implement and operate the systems initially and for the long term fruitfully. Investigating zoning regulations will become a necessity for all structures and provide more job opportunities too.

Electrical workers with courage and experience demonstrate the necessity of artificial intelligence integration with electrical engineering, in addition to the need for hard working blue-collar industrial professionals. There will be a need for exceptional, extremely experienced, and courageous workers. From 6011 to 7018 welding rods, welders will have unimaginable job growth opportunities. Mechanics, plumbers, heating and HVAC experts, and other industrial laborers of all sorts will have bountiful opportunities for existence in a job market that should provide exponential growth opportunities with each and every step taken. There must be quality in everything, and in everything, quality must count. From chimneys to gutters to pipeline creation, as well as formations of all types of new infrastructure and substantial new industries and industrial growth, all will have to be licensed, bonded, and insured moving forward to ensure everything is top notch from the beginning. This will require precision in solutions and applications of all sorts in all fields.

From gas vapor emissions to wastewater management, there will be a need to eliminate all waste products in a manner that is conducive to protecting the immediate environment without the possibility of contamination and with backups to mitigate any possible problem that could exist. Jobs will be plentiful at every environmental learning center, as industrial furnace, wastewater recycling, and food distribution workers, as well as many other industrial professionals, will be needed. The employment opportunities will be bountiful. Employees in these new jobs may become the industry leaders of new fields tomorrow.

The innovations necessary to succeed will also provide amazing opportunities for effective use for mainstream services for mainland use as well, as most will be adaptable and much more efficient than what currently exists in most areas in the world today. Wherever possible, these systems should be integrated into daily usage. Due to adaptability necessities currently still being created, reeducation will be necessary in most cases and in most disciplines. Even travel will be different with more utilization of little transport vehicles like go-karts, self-propelled vehicles, motorized bicycles, and scooters, as they will provide a more comprehensive ability to satisfy travel and parking requirements than traditional methodologies at most of these environmental learning center locations.

Heating, ventilation, and air conditioning, as well as furnace fuel and other sources of energy, will be necessitated differently in each environmental learning center. Job opportunities in these fields will be plentiful, as people like to be cold in the summer and hot in the winter. There is always a need for the person willing to go into the hot attic to create the system. Artificial intelligence will work in a symbiotic relationship with HVAC professionals in creating new highly efficient systems for the future that will be adaptable to numerous environments. These new systems will transform the abilities of efficient energy usage in homes, buildings, and even in the future of spacecraft development. Heating and cooling solutions and methodologies used to create and operate these new systems effectively will provide numerous transformative opportunities, including in maintaining and controlling the amount of enterprising quality improvement enhancements for all people on the planet.

What dictates needs, distribution, and even energy sources themselves will be based on what is realistic and safe for the immediate environment and what can be done safely at the time of implementation. Power components will come in all different forms and will be regulated by both human observation and artificial intelligence monitoring. Water treatment will be necessary for clean drinking water at most of these facilities as well. Wastewater management will be a necessity and may provide its own form of reusable energy eventually; if that is impossible initially, that will have to be accepted temporarily.

The environmental learning centers will need a foremost player in the field of aviation when it comes to lighting runways and other contemplations, as such considerations are also going to play a major role in the expansion of the operational opportunities provided at these facilities. It is possible that, by helping to provide airfield ground lighting, scientific research and development that may enhance opportunities for infrastructure growth at the environmental learning centers, those same developments may be used for lighting enhancement technologies applied on the mainland for more efficient energy expenditure. Air traffic controllers for drones will be necessary during inspection and creation processes, as well as afterwards, for all possible air traffic requirements. Artificial intelligence will enhance the efficiency of the environment and improve the experience in all realms, including avionics.

New findings will also create new fields of study and even more new employment opportunities and should be considered critical to success and always evaluated. As foundational questions emerge, there will need to be justification for what is and has been developed for the promotion of newly adopted concepts of what provides the most realistic opportunities for success for the future of all people and possibilities. OCEM, operational customer experience management, will also be constantly used throughout the creation process and afterwards to give real time feedback to provide a blueprint for greater transparency on how effectively things are operating.

Programs for agriculture and agrarian studies are intrinsically essential for success. Fields such as marine biology and engineering may become included in the college educational program for undergraduate tuition costs in the future as well. We may one day look at marine biologists as doctors of the oceans and farmers as doctors of the land. Engineering abilities may actually become a prerequisite for becoming a doctor or veterinarian moving forward, depending on implications resulting from the implementation of new abilities and instrumentation, especially as new advents become available.

The building of these self-sustainable residential environments will mean that there should be an expectation for cost-of-living adjustments for inhabitants. The exploration for finding the proper location for each residential environment will take a lot of time and effort. There will be considerable forethought given due to the extreme nature of risks inherent in creating such an environment. People skilled in using remotely controlled drones will be part of a new, burgeoning job market. The experience necessitates using such methodologies to successfully understand what it will take to undertake the construction of each environmental learning center. Qualifications necessary for safeguarding the security of the environment and all inhabitants will be established and adhered to in all practices. As such, evacuation procedures will be necessary for each facility, as well as plans for any other security needs.

Viewpoints can be restricted to queries and enhance opportunities provided by people with knowledge, training, resources, financial management experience, qualifications, work experience, past performance, professional experience in a specific field of study, an understanding of participation requirements, and qualifications for working in management to distinguish between potential growth opportunities and ideas that may lead to unforeseen consequences. From time to time, ideas may be submitted to a government board of directors to work in conjunction with people working with aesthetic qualities to enhance their ability to provide useful feedback. Certain necessities of reality should always prevail in a commonsense fashion of practical application for both construction and maintenance of all facilities. Experts in a field who have ideas to offer should also be appreciated. This is where a nine member board of leadership, such as discussed in all for one and one for all, will be necessitated. This will also provide an excellent opportunity to provide additional structures of guidance using the same premise with a multitude of various necessary fields of application. Multiple such boards may exist, all reporting to a managing board of health.

Companies wishing to partake by participating in any business for either construction or maintenance, any industry wishing to participate in operating a day to day business, or any organization that will function as a business incorporated within the established structure must comply with the highest standards of business practices while performing within the guidelines of stakeholder governance and demonstrating that they are committed to doing business in an appropriate alternative altruistic manner by adhering to guidelines of stakeholder governance where appropriately qualified representatives contribute to the governance direction required under the direction of qualified government representatives governing stakeholder governance qualifications under the framework and guidance held by the various national organizations qualified to participate effectively pursuant to various established national and international evaluation organizations under the framework of the classification created by the Clean the Universe Economy government under the established framework of the provisions of the guidelines provided by the United States government under the direction of the Clean the Universe Economy.

Regulations for zoning requirements will be structured following similar guidelines to the framework currently proposed by the American Land Trade Association. The zoning process will be a very important part of the evaluation process, with appropriate amendments available across the jurisdiction becoming a necessary foundation for development. These environmental learning centers will be in harsh locations where maintaining safety will be a difficult task to begin with. The point will be to help the planet, not to cause frustration and exacerbate damage to an enigmatic, volatile environment. Safety will be a vital necessity.

Actions back words into becoming reality. Showing up is the first step on the road to success in any environment or endeavor. The first thing that is necessary is people with the courage, drive, dedication, and purpose to show up with conviction and create each of these inhabited self-sustaining structures to develop initially and grow substantially in the long term as well. From vegetation to inhabitation to evacuation, all things need to be created.

For these ocean, desert, and volcanic environmental study centers to operate, with security and safety paramount in importance as accidents happen, evacuation contingency plans are necessary. Emergency rescue vehicles, entrance system solutions, temporary housing accommodations, and communication are other necessary considerations. Emergency sprinkler systems and other logistics need planning, in addition to the provision of examples of activities and equipment required for safety and maintenance.

Simple logistical opportunities and operational procedures are necessary for all things, even how to refrigerate milk and deliver corresponding requirements for home and commercial operations. Electricity, the creation of water delivery for indoor plumbing systems, and sewer operations for evacuated digestion products will be compulsory. Additional waste not able to be repurposed for energy creation will be part of a system that leads to mass septic receptacles that are easily emptied into cargo ships or trucks for any excess waste products that need to be removed from the premises. Porta-potties and other waste element removal devices, such as dumpsters, will need to be addressed. Appropriate measures will need to be instituted in all phases of all systems for proper handling.

Greenhouses and other farming will take place directly on the island to help support health, wellbeing, lower costs, and provide food capabilities, including foods from around the world, to ensure food availability even in times of potentially difficult food shortages. Everything from fruit trees to year-round cultivation processes will be instrumental in producing a cost-effective value for food distribution and providing problem protection. Powdered milk and other condensed foods, with minimal preservatives added, that need little additional processing time will be required and maintained for a necessary occasion.

All actions approved and implemented must support surety and accuracy of all information acquired in advance of the creation of each structure to ensure the proper ability to provide safety and good health monitoring. Carpenters and contractors are going to be needed, as are electricians and plumbers. As masons build, we will need to always measure our accuracy. From resonance, hydro levels, and combustion to control solutions, many faces of creation will determine how far each structure will be able to grow to produce remedy and aid after successfully monitoring and receiving knowledge from different educational approaches and applications. Integrated solutions are always necessary as knowledge is accumulated. Ecosystem evolution is inevitable, so, as such, building and maintaining all environmental learning centers must be a malleable process both in thought and actions. From the initial phase of creation and after, we must always be able to adapt accordingly.

Every developed structure will eventually need extensive fiberoptic networks that permit people and artificial intelligence the ability to monitor both internal and external pressure forces and all other applicable data that need to be applied to each structure for safety and prevention, as well as for any other unforeseen complications that may arise. This will ensure complete monitoring of all necessary data and permit data accumulation for purposes of further study, maintenance, and creation, too. Fiberoptic communications may be utilized through the following form, where transponders are used by everyone for all things from different networks, including identification of each individual, classifications of industries, classroom education, training, traveling conditions, text messaging, merchandise payment strategies, life enhancement applications, health monitoring, and much more.

Transport logistics will be well thought out in advance; even so, as with other parts of this endeavor, traffic jams and bumps in the road will occur occasionally. Ships and trucks will be responsible for most deliveries and transportation needs initially. Scooters, bicycles, and mopeds will be the preferred means of transportation on the research island sites built. Motorcycles may be permitted under certain circumstances. It will be very difficult to accommodate passengers, although some visiting passenger vehicles may be required to qualify under certain circumstances. Ambulatory services may also be eligible for exceptional recognition. Four-wheel all-terrain vehicles may also become available and even be utilized as replacement vehicles for school buses and ambulances. Other amenities that are necessary initially may include having the students' teachers also be the people responsible for picking up and bringing children to their classrooms and homes every day.

Twenty-four-hour emergency response capabilities, including emergency personnel, will be necessary at all locations. This will include emergency evacuation logistical information containing full evacuation procedures, emergency response authorities, emergency evacuation locations, emergency response services, including search and rescue personnel, search and rescue vehicles, emergency services vehicles, including ambulatory services vehicles fitted with all necessary equipment fitting the geographic requirements of each specific location, helicopters, and all other necessary amenities and facilities. Airports, even for evacuation purposes, may prove to not be feasible in every location of each facility. Viability will increase with improvements in designs of aircraft and airports.

Communication technology is important and also a major part of the troublesome technological developments necessary to accomplish business and personal goals on these facilities. Cell phone technology is already capable of transmitting text messages as if they were being sent from a satellite phone. The question of range for telephonic communications is still a matter of development and frustration. Towers will need to be constructed in a safe manner. For some locations, satellite phones will be necessary to communicate upon arrival for the foreseeable future. Systems for both intra and interpersonal communication for inhabitants of each structure will need to be addressed.

Unlimited international job growth will exist due to the creation of multiple environmental learning centers, and this should create a consistent demand for new employees for a considerable amount of time, hopefully forever. It is important to recognize that all these advantages and disadvantages we currently face will prepare us for an unknown future where we will be able to bring many of these intellectually challenging creations of necessity back to the mainstream for use in cities and towns throughout the world. The aqueducts and pipelines of yesterday will be replaced with new, efficient, safe technology. All industries and all fields of endeavor will see significant improvements in functionality. This will lead to further employment opportunities and then interplanetary opportunities in the future. These disadvantages of today will promote our necessity to create answers, and those learners that we meet along the way will help us to understand ourselves and the mysteries of the galaxies and our Universe. These centers will become the new testing grounds and provide the requisite templates we shall need for maximizing our abilities to successfully inhabit other planets in the future. These centers will provide the necessary education for human beings to be able to know how to make an uninhabitable planet a new home. Every success starts with taking the first step; the time is now. Soon, we shall need to celebrate our achievements and accomplishments with a major international celebration and day of appreciation that is illustrious as a day of world heritage for all.

Eventually, each environmental learning center will be a prime alpha reflection service market in many industries, with an emphasis placed on future generations with thriving bakeries, restaurants, the food service industry, hotels and coffee shops. Entrepreneurs with adventurous spirits will be required to meet eligibility requirements. From mom-and-dad run shops to big box stores, all will have a niche to fill within the ability to provide goods and services to a variety of different populations and to fit geographical locational limitations.

Every facility will have its own fields for baseball, soccer, and softball, a golf course, as well as pickleball, basketball and tennis courts for all inhabitants of each center to participate in health-related recreational activities. Artificial surfaces may be a necessity in certain geographic locations. There will be fields and services for the physically and mentally healthy, as well as those who need assistance, including Little League fields for children built to Miracle League specifications. Sports serve as a reminder of health and wellbeing. There is an intrinsic value that brings enrichment and fulfillment to those who are involved in participating in something larger than themselves. Positive social interactions and interpersonal communications are all enhanced by involvement in healthy activities.

We are all registered to volunteer at any place and at any time. All individuals have the right to help each other. Volunteers will qualify for tax reductions or school credits when not reimbursed. This situation may be beneficial in terms of how to meet the needs of qualified professionals in certain areas until supplemental staff can be educated. These volunteer initiatives will be across the spectrum of volunteer opportunities and, in areas like education, will require volunteers to meet regularly during the recruitment process, as well as meet quarterly qualifications afterwards.

Every individual member of the environmental learning centers is responsible for maintaining civility and providing discourse for the necessary regulations to form a basis that permits cohesive conduct of the collective. Volunteers will be notified of what psychological barriers may inevitably be detrimental to long-term health, and nutrition guidelines will also be established. The day and age of taking advantage of those with less education or cognitive abilities will no longer be tolerated. There needs to be proper program management within a core covenant agreement that the truth and what is best for life to exist optimally shall be the deciding factors of behavior and choices. Accomplishing our prime objectives shall lead to eliminating potential opportunities for corruption that often negatively impact the quality of life. The removal of exploitation will enhance all of our knowledge quality management efforts. This will result in a better landscape of health for all involved at all levels of the environmental learning centers. A declaration of human rights that serves as a foundational centerpiece of decency will be formed. Under this core covenant, agreed to by any and all participants, adherence is mandatory for continued involvement with each and every one of the environmental learning centers. This will include eventual intergenerational engagement between key stakeholders such as government representatives, investors, and contributors of all levels, including familial participants.

Members of the environmental learning centers should demonstrate pride in, and a commitment to, creating infrastructure solutions for generations with a concentration on local development dedicated to industrial infrastructure utilizing independent and government contractors in a coordinated, cohesive covenant of creation where safety and ingenuity are required. From the days of John Oldham and even in the spirit of Oldham, England, it has always been necessary to exhibit appreciation for doing the difficult things required for survival and thriving. While we cannot be too rigid, quality control monitoring is a necessity. We must be flexible and allow the road ahead to tell us when, where, and even how we will inevitably succeed totally.

How many degrees of California thermal requirements have actually been useful in helping to preserve or improve the natural environment? It is time for actual action that provides actual positive results. It is time for us to consider the fact that health for ourselves as a whole requires a healthy planet as well. While these things may seem astonishing, they will lead us into a wonderful tomorrow immediately. Maybe Andre the Giant visited Petra, the Taj Mahal, Chichen Itza, Machu Picchu, Christ the Redeemer, the Colosseum, and the Great Wall of China; maybe not. Either way, we are going to find things that are even more wondrous in our explorations on our planet, in our oceans, in spacc, and eventually on other planets.

Do not listen to the peanut gallery telling us all the negatives that might transpire. Instead, let us find ourselves in the middle by creating a positive future for existence for all of us forever. The days may seem dark now; however, we shall embrace the path ahead, creating our own luminosity that brightens the prospects that lie in wait for all of us on the distant horizon of tomorrow. We shall keep our blinders on when necessary and always have confidence that it will always be worth it, for the light at the end of the tunnel will be amazing and awesome.

CHAPTER 9

GOVERNANCE

The precursor to the Declaration of Independence and the Constitution of the United States of America served as an antecedent for the phrase "We the People" as well as the inalienable, self-evident right for each citizen to be endowed with the pursuit of happiness. In fact, this initial, mostly forgotten document of important resolves provided many of the sentiments that would be displayed in the document written by Thomas Jefferson with the aid, assistance, and worldly knowledge accumulated by Benjamin Franklin. Encouragement for Jefferson's writings also came in the form of another future president with very different ideas: John Adams. This long overlooked historical script would also serve to provide the basis of the formation of the government of the United States of America as well. The initial document that these men drew upon is known as the Sheffield Declaration, written by farmers in Sheffield, Massachusetts. The town meeting in Sheffield on January 12, 1773, was the original conception for the country of the United States of America that was labored upon and born on July 2, 1776, adopted on July 4, 1776, and signed on August 2, 1776. Many of the ideals that led to a revolution are present within. One of the resolves of the Sheffield Declaration states, "Mankind in a state of nature are equal, free, and independent of each other, and have a right to the undisturbed enjoyment of their lives, their liberty and property."

The proof that we are supposed to care about all in the United States in our basic documents of government is shown by the very fact that the words "We the People" are the first three words of the preamble of the United States Constitution. This determined the path that the United States would be for and by the people as a more perfect, tranquil union that would be administered by a government that was run by the people in all phases of the decision-making process. While seemingly not always demonstrated, all those who govern in the United States of America have a responsibility to the people. The power of the United States of America lies with its citizenry. "We the People" will always be the first words written to stand for freedom for all people. We are for the people, by the people, and that is the meaning behind the flag of the United States and what it stands for, shields, and protects.

Further proof that we, the citizens of the United States of America, are supposed to care about all in the United States is straightforward in our regime's documents. This concept is shown by the Constitution of the United States in the very fact that we are formed as a republic and not a democracy. What is the main difference between a democracy and a republic? In a democracy the minority view is not allowed to express itself publicly all the time, if at all. The United States takes the minority viewpoint to the relevance it deserves by providing a basis for hearing and understanding, even in our Supreme Court cases, so that the merit of the argument is understood from both the majority and minority viewpoints.

The United States is shown to be a democratic republic, and the Constitution is the document that, when acted upon by We the People, guarantees this as the form of government that is utilized. This creates a foundation for all portions of the Constitution to be implemented and maintained. With this new program, we will be bringing government to be thought of as a positive entity and a good thing for and by all the people of our country and hopefully in other countries, too. When these effects are brought to fruition, the lives that they will encourage will help all of us to evolve in life for and by all of the people.

Providing a cut above with our elected officials so that we can have the most altruistic intelligence is a long overdue necessity in our political landscape. Leadership in our government should be where knowledge and kindness prevail in each application. This is a necessity for good governance. While difficult in certain instances, leadership in a position of authority over a particular population propagated in its situation by financial growth and where information influences decisions requires inherent honor in all phases of guidance. The best teams are the ones that have the best management in all facets. The battle of moral integrity should not be one forgotten; it should be the point for all of us and all life.

As a member of We the People, as a citizen of the United States, do right by taking responsibility for your actions and for various initiatives of industrial governance. Be as effective as possible in being as exact as imaginable so that the road to the eradication of errors is narrowed substantially. We must do so in the attempt to eliminate any concerning consequences resulting from unforeseen variations from the predictive model analysis provided previously by detailed logistical forecasts on how to be successful. This will be exhibited in the years ahead by a methodical communication model created by a systematic symbiotic relationship between artificial and human intelligence and from all levels of available material from any source of information that is willing to contribute to life and health.

In order to be effective, enabling self-governance has to precede governance by a doctor, let alone governance by the state. One must be able to regulate oneself and understand how to apply and take action for necessitated evolution before being capable of accepting such instruction from an outside source, especially if action is also required. One of the most simple forms of maturation that people often demonstrate within their own lives is when they start to incorporate the concept of need versus want in their daily lives. Understanding that food must be available, gas for the car is needed, electricity helps to keep us functional, and heat is necessary to survive in the winter is not glamorous, yet these concepts make up most people's day-to-day realities of necessity for maintaining life.

For the individual to live a healthy life for as long as possible, becoming as good as possible at understanding this concept helps tremendously. For the rare few who do not need to be concerned with such things, they are fortunate to not have to make as many sacrifices to simply exist on a day-to-day basis to be able to just continue to do so, especially if they do not need to sacrifice want for familial need. For the vast majority of the populace of the United States and the world, though, that is not reality. The reality is that simply needing to survive is a prerequisite in order to be able to have any chance of ever being able to thrive.

This concept is often found to be true for the rearing of a child by a parent. Most good parents will tell you that, as parents, they have often had to sacrifice what they wanted as individuals for the sake of what is good for their children. This noble concept of parental sacrifice used to be the norm; however, now it appears that such good intentions should not be taken for granted. The greatest gift in life is time; especially quality time well spent. The only gift greater is life itself. Giving life and then helping that person to grow to one day become a positive being in his or her own right is and always will be the most important purpose of existence because, without that action, existence ceases to exist. The propagation and perpetuation of the species depend on such a concept for the ability to discover the hope of tomorrow's promise of possibilities.

This concept of self-governance is relevant for each of us as individuals and possibly as parents, and it is the same notion that also expands to our town and local governments, too. This is true for us as individuals before even arriving at how such a concept works on state administrative and federal government levels as well. Governments should also be concerned with what people need over what people want. This is the basis of infrastructure. Proper allocation of resources on an efficient basis is always part of good governance. This is especially true when budgets are limited, and, often, most constituencies do not want to be concerned with the government saving money for a necessary project tomorrow when those funds may be returned to them as individual taxpayers today.

There appears to be incredible angst and consternation demonstrated over which political party seems to be representing a person's values the most these days. This is strange, as many of the people on both sides have apparently joined the same secret societies in the past, and many of these government bureaucrats may also have the same hidden agendas even though they are on opposite sides of the aisle. Often, there are jokes created by truth that many of these elected officials attend the same functions and frequently associate with the same people as their supposed opposition does as well. It is of vital importance that we, the people, as individuals and also as a collective, do not get distracted by the show.

In regard to contemplating whom to vote for, it would be logical for most people to ask the question: Do the policies of the person who is running for office help the average middle-class citizen? Most federal financial policies that have been introduced for the past couple of decades have come at the expense of the middle class and have shut down most mom and pop owned businesses around the country. The days of Main Street have been replaced by the big box store, and now small business owners of all sorts, and even several big box stores, are being pushed out of business in favor of major conglomerate corporations. It seems that the vast majority of government officials only care about winning the next election, not leading. The reality, on both the Democratic and Republican sides, is that the rich keep getting richer and the average citizen is being taken advantage of in order to do so. Fortunately, there are people in leadership on both sides who are trying to stop fraud and do good deeds every day, which is difficult given the circumstances, because there are many people who do not want to lose their power by any means. Meanwhile, the American people are divided purposely so that they do not stand together against the corruption.

In reality, high minimum wages do not help most communities or the country. While high minimum wages are theoretically helpful, the actuality is that most small business owners cannot afford to stay in business after such wages are introduced. In addition to paying their staff higher wages, small business owners also have to pay increased health insurance premium rates, resulting in additional overhead cost expenditures. Also, there have been rules put into place by the federal government and several state governments about the number of people who work for a company, resulting in the need for various levels of health insurance options. This has resulted in even big box stores not offering enough hours for their employees to qualify as full time to be eligible for health insurance. Smaller business owners generally do not have the ability to afford the staff to circumvent the same policies. All of this has created an untenable financial situation for many small, midsize, and intermediate business owners, which makes it difficult, if not impossible, to stay in business. The market must be able to bear the cost. Acceptable minimum wage standards vary by state and depend on cost-of-living indexes, which vary dramatically geographically. Waste, fraud, and abuse need to be cleared up in every state to truly understand the necessary information to formulate a genuine financial index for the actual cost of living in different regions to have realistic calculations that are based on authenticity for each state's population. The policies being forced now in relation to minimum wage just close the door permanently on small and intermediate size business owners and have shut the door, it seems, permanently on the American Dream for most.

Problems with consolidated power exist within governments and within corporations that are becoming monopolies, and such problems may even be the cause of conflict in local communities as well as in neighboring states. Societies can be overrun by personal ambitions versus what the population actually votes for and wants. When small factions take power over the vast majority of societal networks, it can create a substantial problem where what is being done is actually the exact opposite of what was wanted or intended by the massive mainstream.

In many industries, there appears to be a consolidation of the marketplace occurring. While the big box stores took over Main Street previously, many of those big box stores have now fallen to the wayside as well. The merging of various companies into major conglomerates is something that keeps coming up routinely in federal investigations. The rule against monopolies is being tested, if not bested, in many cases, and this erodes financial viability.

There is a major sports network that is buying up the rights to all types of sports that used to have their own forms of broadcast or online presence. A lack of viable alternatives for broadcasting is now leading teams in some significant leagues to put all of their broadcasts under the same company umbrella. This is also happening in Hollywood, where very powerful production companies that have been famous for years are now being bought up by the same company that used to have a completely different design and platform of operations. These mega-conglomerates now have incredible control over their originally intended marketplaces and also generally have branched out into ownership of other significant companies in different industries and may even be multinational as well. Too much influence on a major international level or on a local scale is not usually a healthy environment for most people. Power may become an impediment to innovative solutions.

Town managers have been guilty in certain circumstances of ruining towns by doing what is best in the short term and kicking the can down the road with real problems. This has been done by many town managers so that their own reputations are enhanced for future jobs in other towns they hope to go manage elsewhere someday. Sometimes now, town managers do not even live in the town they are managing and do not feel the burden of their own policy creations. In addition, the methodologies used by certain town managers may not show the true will of the people living in that town.

Circumventing votes by the town citizenry by holding meetings in areas too small to accommodate everyone, with crowds too large for anyone to be heard or recognized, has become commonplace. Constantly, it is the elderly in town who have the most difficulty in attending such meetings, let alone being recognized, and often they are the largest taxpayers in a town. The town will often claim this system works as well as voting, despite many people in attendance being left feeling as though it was almost impossible for anyone to be heard at the town meeting. Holding meetings in venues that are overcrowded, do not have adequate parking, and are often nearly impossible for the elderly, infirm, and handicapped to access or to traverse to be able to be recognized and heard from is a serious problem.

These meetings will often occur when an idea is being pushed through to avoid the possibility of the town inhabitants voting down the concept and not approving it. Unfortunately, this is also done purposely to create large pools of money to be used for pilfering and embezzlement. Quite often, school systems are used for these purposes. If the intent was really the education of the children, then why is it so often found that the creation of schools costs a fortune, and yet the children still have courses currently removed from the opportunities available to them?

Worse yet, after the meeting, sometimes other agendas are introduced. This may lead to an increase in taxes on other matters that may not have anything to do with items discussed in the meeting. An example of this is holding a meeting for a new school and then, after forcing approval of the new school, sending out letters about how water mains and roads need immediate repairs, so taxes will be increased further. This is even more egregious when it is done through a false implication that the road matter has been discussed at some point previously in past discussions and through mailings that may have never actually been sent out at any point before the actual letter in question arrives. Pretending that increases have been the subject of conversation before they are actually discussed is a form of fraud. The town may then raise taxes even more on the citizenry for other essential items, such as water supplies, sewage disposal, town road repaving, and other necessary items, such as street signs, stoplights, snow plowing, salt, sand, snow removal, and the development of other infrastructure needs. While residents surely will appreciate these necessary services, each member of the local community needs to have the ability to decide what other materials and matters should be included in what their taxpayer money is going to be spent upon in the town's yearly budget.

In 1215, the Magna Carta was created as society made it clear that even the king is not above the people; in fact, all people are responsible for their actions. Even the king is a member of the people, never above the people. It is the responsibility of the king, or any system of governance, to make sure that the safety of the people, the wellbeing of the people, the security of the people, and the needs of the people are satisfactorily met to the best of the leadership's ability. This needs to always be done in an ethical environment that promotes the health and wellbeing of all of the citizens, not some, but all of the citizens.

The king's job, as it should be in any system of government responsible for the multitudes, is to feed the needs of all the people, not to have the king's ego fed. If that is not the case, the king will lose his crown, or the system of government will cease to function successfully if it continues to operate at all. This is also the problem when governments lose their way of working in a collective core covenant always united for and about the citizens. This is what occurs when politics becomes more important than providing a fundamental system of government that works for all individuals. Governance is more important than politics because government is ideally for all the people and helps any person who is affected by that leadership's plan, while politics only works for the citizens who believe in that political system of management. This is not the time for some; this is the time for all, and all means all. Once again, not some, all means all, quite literally, and should be that way forever.

Successful governments operate in a pragmatic and practical fashion that meets the needs of the citizens of that country, government and geographic location. Officials of a regime have a responsibility to provide the resources necessary specifically for their people and should do so in a national government that operates efficiently and effectively for the citizens affected by that administration. No other country or entity should interfere with the success of another country being run in such a way that the people are prospering well.

There have been instances of severe political discord that have influenced politics and government in the United States of America for at least the past thirty years, if not since our inception. When it comes to international relations and diplomacy, these unfortunate disputes have prevented people and companies from thriving as much as possible and have served, to a significant degree, to form a lack of coherence in how to move forward collaboratively. The direction of vitriolic anger on a personal level has served to create an atmosphere of distrust, disloyalty, dislike and to dismantle the fabric of the integrity of our nation. What began as investigations turned into impeachment proceedings both in the 1990s and, as we have witnessed recently, with our current president. Neither now nor then have any of these actions, statements, and acerbic harassment helped. This lack of cohesion has manifested into a much larger problem and has led to a culture of violence and attempts at assassination. This negativity has laid the foundation of a society that is fighting against itself instead of endeavoring to build a better tomorrow together today.

We cannot continue to proceed like this. We need to do better for ourselves, our children, and for all people alive today and in the future. Whether it be a Democrat, Republican, or possibly a candidate from another party in the future of the United States of America, we must respect the office of the presidency even if we do not respect the person who is president. We must always remain loyal with absolute integrity to the governing power that counts the most in all ways because that always has been and always will be we, the people.

The innate individual interest in political ideology creates an opportunity for the perversion of one's inherently intimate involvement with any form of government to feel trampled upon. This may lead to the destruction of the environment of trust and integrity that is necessary for the protection of the people and for any possibility of having an opportunity to participate in something larger than ourselves. Disagreements about the direction of leadership should be made in a manner of respect out of the responsibilities that are necessary to provide effective leadership for our communities, municipalities, counties, districts, current regimes, future establishments of leadership, and especially our country.

Different governments work well with different governmental structures and systems. This concept and reality should definitively contribute to how we function together moving forward. There are good reasons why diverse administrations are suited and needed for different regimes, from unalike generations of struggling to even geographically dissimilar countries. The various unique challenges that are presented demonstrate that different methodologies are required to meet the needs of the population in each individual country.

Country involvement in the Clean the Universe program should be operational in the same way that federalism currently works within the United States. We have an opportunity to find ways to successfully implement our program if we are able to maintain our independence from one another as countries and still work together to accommodate the realities of each other as one team united in the concept of a collective responsibility in order to achieve a healthy global perspective. Every nation will choose which government works best for that individual country and the people of that land. Each nation will do so in a manner that provides the necessary basis for sustainable success of the environmental learning centers and for the collective population of the world.

Not every foundation is expected to be identical. As such, we should not expect every institution to look the same. Even from an equal basis, different ideologies and premises of perfection may be exceptionally different from person to person. What works today may not work tomorrow, so finding success requires constant adaptation over the ages of time. Sometimes, though, the same foundation may be used successfully throughout many eras.

Heidelberg Castle in Germany is associated with being a residence for maneuvering and shaping the evolution of Europe over the course of history for many centuries. Only part of the foundation of Heidelberg Castle has been rebuilt since the seventeenth and eighteenth centuries. Since its original creation in the year 1214, it became two castles in 1294 and then one castle again after a lightning strike in 1537. The castle has held up after being involved in invasions, being set on fire, being blown up with mines, and even facing just the threat of age over time. The natural decay that has occurred has threatened the existence of the castle's foundations, but they are still there. Even in this instance, where the same foundation has been utilized time and time again, what has been built upon it was for success during the period of creating the structures necessary for survival. With time, while what is built needs to adapt, the foundation should remain unchanged when it serves the needs of the population.

Just as not every government should operate in the same environment and not every federal government should run the same, not every household and family should operate in the same environment and fashion. Whatever works best is something that needs to be determined on an individual basis with intensely intimate knowledge of the environment in question. There should be no gerrymandering. Governor Elbridge Gerry of Massachusetts, a signer of the Declaration of Independence, personally did not like the practice of gerrymandering and found it to be "highly disagreeable." All elections should be done by county with no manipulation of geographical areas. The local inhabitants know what works best for them based on the realities of where they live, not some nonsensical lines drawn on a map.

Regarding the environmental learning centers, pro-jurisdictional requirements will be reviewed quarterly and annually for all participants in the program to make sure that they are complying with all regulations necessary for involvement. For the people of countries where individuals live without constitutional protection, as well as for those people who live freely already, the environmental learning centers are meant to assist all people for the rest of time. A unified cooperation forged through peace means these conditions may make the difference between survival and not being able to find any hope for the next generation. Consistency in action after beginning will be even more important than during the initial implementation to avoid false promises, opportunities for corruption, and negative influences.

Many of the issues we are dealing with today are not necessarily new at all; other matters are extraordinarily new. In fact, looking back on thousands of years, societal concerns for millions of individuals are very similar to those of bygone epochs; however, how quickly the ramifications may be felt by society and the degree to which they may impact civilization are exceptionally different than in past millennia. An example of this is that people still need to eat and have warmth when it is cold, although the methodologies employed for doing these things are vastly different now than in past centuries and eras. The reality is that the world is very different due to the power we have achieved, especially over the past one hundred and twenty-five years as well. War was once fought with rocks, bows, and arrows; now leaders of certain governments have the ability to literally blow up the world. Because of that power, the world is susceptible to corruption and vulnerable to destruction now more than ever before. It is also possible that this devastation can happen faster as well.

Today, an issue may lead to an investigation by an analytical branch of administration through many techniques and technological advancements that did not so readily exist even just a few decades ago. Additionally, government operations are threatened by a shutdown of known surveillance networks more than at any point in history beforehand. Items acknowledged as government online surveillance methods include electronic tools such as mobile phones and televisions, as well as text messages. These apparatuses are technological communications network devices equipped with information detection technology known as online surveillance systems created by law enforcement personnel. These communication equipment devices provide information through multiple quality services such as surveillance cameras, online surveillance, video surveillance, text messaging, and application usage information management, including any online information from a telephone or any other capable electronic communications equipment. All of these data collection methodologies provide knowledge for an investigation. The introduction of these methods has been questioned repeatedly as being overly intrusive into privacy and intimacy.

The significance of the usage of these methods is subject to uncertainty of understanding and imagination, which can lead to catastrophic intended and unintended consequences. This occurs when there is a lack of understanding, ingenuity, and willingness to cooperate. In terms of security, due to possible individual and group threats of mass destruction, we are at a time when the team is far more important than the individual. While this is true, the individual needs to be respected as well. Now, data is frequently collected from people using apps on their phones and online devices, and that collection is authorized by the user as part of the initial agreement to use the application. In these instances, all information gathered should be utilized only for enhancing opportunities and quality of existence for the user and for no other reason. Even when this data is being gathered by a government intelligence agency, it is important to remember that the information collected needs to be kept confidential and used for no purpose other than an ongoing investigation. National implementation of such detective methods leads to quality evaluation questions such as these: What quality improvement options exist?

What opportunities are there for protection of all accumulated information? What occurs with the knowledge garnered? Are there any forms of performance evaluation that are done in an audit fashion after monitoring a person or a company for those involved in the inquiry? What happens to someone's private information moving forward after the initial implementation of such techniques? Who has access to the materials involved later? What happens if the government agency's systems are hacked into after the investigation? Could these same systems be weaponized against the very people who collected the intel? While Section 702 of the Foreign Intelligence Surveillance Act (FISA) has lapsed, the Foreign Intelligence Surveillance Court (FISC) has approved a one-year programmatic certification, legally grandfathering ongoing intelligence collection. Will future legislation concerning the collection of intelligence address these issues that have been mentioned? Will artificial intelligence play a significant role in data collection, security, and intelligence information protection monitoring moving forward?

The first democracy that human beings are presently aware of was created 2,500 years ago in Athens, Greece, and it permitted every free Athenian man who had completed military training the right to have a vote that counted in the assembly. This was the beginning of the realization that it is the average citizen who always gives any government strength. From the day of that first meeting of the assembly until today, this truth is still the reality of how many people feel good about the circumstances of life in regard to government matters in the free world. The ancient Greek people witnessed what works effectively and efficiently, and while they did not follow through far enough, gave birth to the concept that civilians should have power. While the direct democracy of the Athenians is different from the constitutional republic of the United States of America, it is important to remember that the USA has led the way in the significance of the individual and still does. Maintaining the integrity and independence of the free individual is still the basis of the government of the United States. Life, love, liberty and the pursuit of happiness are still essential today.

Like Clovis I, who united all of the Franks into Francia, we will also be permitting different opportunities for government implementation by permitting several languages to be spoken as they were in the time of Charlemagne. As always, this can cause communication complications, such as those in modern day India, where Hindi is spoken in most places, but not everywhere. In most regions of India, individuals initially speak languages that are spoken only in their immediate geographic locations, as the dialects give way to community and demonstrate where people emanate from in the country. Castilian Spanish is like the King's English in being the proper grammatical way of speaking and writing for each language. Another similarity is that no one speaks the King's English or Castilian Spanish in the United States of America. These things lead to communication difficulties when people try to speak to others after learning English or Spanish, and these difficulties are often seen when people learn other languages, too. People are often surprised that learning a foreign language is only the beginning, as it is necessary to learn the dialects and colloquialisms that are actually spoken by most people, which can vary vastly in different regions and territories.

Since the days of Gaul, Gallia Belgica, Gallia Lugdunensis, and Gallia Aquitania were created under the direct supervision and direction of Julius Ceasar and his son Augustus, including the absorption of Gallia Cisalpina into what would become the northern part of the country now called Italy, countries can change. Poland even ceased to exist for one hundred and twenty-three years and then disappeared from the maps of the world once more during and after World War II. Poland truly did not regain its sovereignty again until 1989, when, on the last day of the year, the Polish eagle was once again returned to the country's flag.

The creation of the Senate in ancient Rome has given us the knowledge that there are other important elements of what is necessary to create a system of government that operates effectively and efficiently as well. Such is the necessity of government institutions and the need for proper governance processes. As the world changes, adaptations must be made.

While crossing the Rubicon has come to take on a meaningful definition of finality, it is also a reason to find hope in current circumstances in which hope is hard to find right now. When Julius Ceasar crossed the Rubicon River, it marked the point of no return in what was an impending civil war. While there may not be much to take as a silver lining from that concept regarding current conflicts that have gone on far too long, there actually is one important piece to derive that provides hope now for peace to be found. The fact that this phrase is used by both sides of the unfortunate conflict in the Middle East is actually a sign that these two opposing sides that claim to have nothing in common now are really viewing the whole matter in some ways as a civil war, much like the conflict Julius Ceaser initiated.

That makes it conceivable, by definition, that it possibly means both sides of this unfortunate matter view each other as familiar. Maybe that is why the wounds hurt so much as well. Since civil war is a division of like-minded and similar individuals and cultures, maybe this small but important portion of parallel understanding can invoke the idea of family and be enough of a common point of understanding that it provides an opportunity for future communications of relevance. Maybe, in the future, this will not have the same finality that it is thought to have now, and information may be available that provides for a long overdue, much needed, and inspirational peace accord to be reached immediately. Our differences should be valued; our similarities should be held as sacred.

An area of Los Angeles, California, in the United States of America, is now referred to as Tehrangeles by some. This is an area where Iranian culture is predominant and cultural aspects of Iranian culture, stores, and food are prevalent. In reality, many cultures, including Israeli and other Middle Eastern societies, live in this section of Los Angeles, and it is a wonderful mixture of various people who come from countries that have never really gotten along. Unfortunately, due to recent conflicts, there has been growing tension among members of the public, who are an astounding and outstanding representation of how a positive, peaceful environment can be created by people who share much in common. While many people propagate passionately that there is little fundamentally to be shared by these people in religion or in application of other concepts of truth of God, common ground is found. Peace still reigns supreme through it all, even while there is such unrest elsewhere.

It is possible the long hair of the Merovingians may have been a status symbol of a democratic system of government. At that time in Gaul, long hair was usually only the kind of thing that the king, or even only the tribal leader of the Franks, would have as a status symbol. The Merovingians were apparently different in that they permitted others who would usually be considered subservient to the king to also have a status symbol of that representation, which would indicate a possibility of a government system based on equality, or at least equivalent potential, as a foundation of the structure of their society. At the same time, it may not, but what it does indicate is the prospect that there was some thoughtful consideration being given to how to create equality and a prosperous, healthy tomorrow for all. It would be one of the first moments where equality was demonstrated.

If this plan is ever enacted, the potential for opportunities is endless. A number of programs that could be created will be well subsidized because of people coming off of state aid programs. State support money saved can be used to develop new or enhance existing programs for clothing donations, for the education of children, for the elderly, and for feeding those in need in general. The number of individuals who are unable to carry out activities of daily living will be aided in doing so as well.

All children have the right to have further education regardless of any other circumstances. Water and food need to be provided to all children, no matter what obstacles and conditions need to be overcome. The time is now to find a way to provide clean water, increased oxygen, and vibrant soil for all of the children worldwide without exception. Enough with the excuses. It is important to create a world where all children are able to sleep in a bed at night in a safe and secure manner, knowing they are in a positive, healthy environment.

This program focuses on the ugly duckling becoming the swan. This program provides valuable resources to improve the quality of life for all people along the way to our destination. It provides the opportunity to move forward in a manner that is consistent with our values and beliefs. What does streamlined and individualized really mean? With all components of this program, it means an all-inclusive principle with a custom touch for each individual that is specifically tailored to that particular person's individual needs. It also means that all people have significance in their value.

We will begin our work now and continue to make progress in creating quality time immediately by communicating the layers, textures, and techniques that will be necessary for implementation and continuous improvement. We can only control what we can control, so go with the flow. We shall always aim for perfection in the hopes of achieving excellence, with our mark being that of consistency. Our vision needs to be clearly focused on the importance of implementing this program immediately.

We will work diligently so that the proof of how this effort is to be made becomes easy to see, and with every positive choice, there will be the opportunity for slightly more positive consequences. This will be done consistently with continuity of purpose that allows for an eventually better foundation for choice with positivity tomorrow in all regions of Earth. Once we do this a few times, a few steps from now, even the homeless will have better opportunities and assistance in achieving.

The whole coin is always there, and it needs to be; this is how things actually work and are supposed to in reality. There must be day and night. Pain teaches us to appreciate happiness. Loss is when we realize what we had previously gained. There must be bad to appreciate the good in life. There is a paradoxical nature of existence that is inherently necessary and, mysterious as it may be, a requirement for a healthy environment.

Too much cleaning can be a bad thing as well. Balance is important in recognizing what is worth saving and what you must be willing to move forward from. Completely eviscerating everything is not a healthy way to move forward; it only separates you from where you were, and hence all the evolutional growth that can be inspiring going forward can expire. There are good bacteria and bad bacteria; human beings and most of existence need both forms to survive and have proper equilibrium for life. The answer is not an eradication of one or the other; it is finding the appropriate balance.

This will be a free cleaning, and then we shall save what was cleaned and use it for prosperity, so truth may always be seen for what it was without reinvention of the narrative to fit the script. Then we shall speed to unlimited energy flow leading to a glowing positive impact putting our children first once and for all. This will be done for a synergistic reality mindset to help lessen the gulf between the world that was and the new world that is destined. It is truth found and needs to be accepted for all actions to be relevant afterwards.

Most of the activities that we perform seem incredibly important in the moment, and yet, after that, people may experience a total loss of recollection that they even performed in or were involved in a particular activity. At other times, a person may do things, and those things aesthetically have one significant importance to an individual or assembly, while another person or group may not have any sense of appreciation for that same performance. Most of what we do in life truly can be described as something and nothing. The action taken significantly demonstrates that there was an importance in performing the action initially; however, the lack of recognition or complete lack of recollection is proof that there is not true import shown long term in some instances. Then again, that may be the significance.

Being able to create a society where all people, for the entirety of time, have the ability to be hall of fame participants is more important than ideologies that have been proven to be failures like equity. Equity limits the individual's and the team's ability to achieve. Every athletic hall of fame and all artistic museums are full of the accomplishments of people who discovered a superlative manner to amplify their own innate abilities to prosper by being who they actually authentically are, not some generic variety of another person's prearranged supposition of how an achievement should be performed.

Equity is a terrible concept that prohibits existence. This plan should never have a court of chancery, as equity is doomed to fail because it is inherently a self-defeating prophecy. In the attempt to remove bias, incredible amounts of bias must be introduced, let alone adhered to, in order to initiate and attempt the concept. Equity inevitably leads to the realization that to help some, more than those initially affected, must be harmed. Equality is a good thing for all; equity kills all. Equality is created with this plan for all people forever.

Living in a free society of competition permits the ability to be for good for real, not just in theory. The difference is massive in its results. Those who stand for a redistribution of wealth generally do so from a position where it benefits them specifically over the masses, which belies the intention of the concept and proves that those undertaking such an endeavor are hypocrites who are selfish.

The big, bright, beautiful community that we are able to create, one that is full of wonder, promise, harmony, bliss, and evolving hearts, is real, possible, and there for the taking; however, it is important to do so in a manner that actually works, not with theories that do not and prove to be counterproductive in time. If we find that there are other sources of disruption that are negatively impacting the willingness it takes to succeed, then these sources of disruption should be examined and, if possible, strengthened, and, if not, examined for another alternative answer for potential implications and implementation.

Unlimited artisans grant more opportunities to meet any obstacle with persistence and original creative thought patterns, which empower doing good, right valued actions. We will do so with a financial mindset of always having right on the money value, allowing us to spruce our efforts and, through proper enforcement, pursue our lofty ambitions of creating a permanent environment conducive to natural wellness and health for all of us.

Being the sentry and being the good shepherd are not concepts of theory; they are proven only through the realization of actions that lead directly to positive results. Only our actions count, not our theories. Take care of your immediate environment, mow your lawn, edge your property, grow flowers, and clean up the trash around your yard. If you see garbage on the ground next to where you happen to be at that moment in time, pick it up and throw it out. Use those extra gloves from Covid to remove trash in your neighborhood and surrounding area, as doing so may provide benefits of unforeseen positivity in your own community.

Why is there no blame being placed on past or present occurrences? When the doctor arrives at the emergency room, determining fault is not apposite; only immediately providing a remedy with the appropriate application of care is suitable, so that health may return. Gentle kindness, beginning with honesty with ourselves, and appreciation for our own existence take each of us much further in the journey of life.

It will take time and patience to see the total fruition of our labors. If success is readily apparent much faster than anticipated or expected, it can still take a while for people to get adjusted to new surroundings and concepts. Even under the best of conditions, it can take weeks for the human mind to accomplish having our individual circadian rhythms adjusted to any new situation or circumstances. It may even take a long time thereafter for the human body to be able to adjust to new settings and environments.

A passing of the torch means understanding a generational approach of positivity in some ways reminiscent of the prorogation of Parliament and what transpires after a session of achievement. The evolution of ideas was even prevalent in the creation of the United States when the

Church of England made alterations to their public mindset in 1713 that were part of what led to revolution in 1776. Beforehand, with the revival of plays in 1660, Thespis' performances helped encourage the reform of England, bringing an end to the days of Puritanism and possibly leading directly to banking changes and, at the very least, contributing to a societal environmental overhaul of true significance.

From when Nathan Hale commenced the inception of our Union, giving the only life he had for the United States of America to be born, through moments of internal unrest such as Shays' Rebellion and other core issues of divide, people like George Washington and Abraham Lincoln have been keeping the world in motion with passion so we positively prevail powerfully on our promise, maintaining the tranquility of our Union. It is important that we protect the right to pursue happiness just as they did. We must find courage like Hale, have the conviction of Shays, display the resolve of Lincoln, and create like Washington so we may keep the world in motion with passionate positive purpose of action. In doing so, we will be doing God's work together as an all-faith congregation of one.

Honest, open, and willing to listen, that is how we can commence and continue with this concept, every one of us feeling every moment, every sensation, and allowing ourselves to accept. From a perspective of health, happiness, and fulfillment, there are sunny days ahead. We shall be the seeds of health and positivity; we just need to add our planet's clean water with a breath of fresh air. The legacy we leave behind shall be one of friendly worldwide goodwill with a refreshing perspective and the ability to hit high notes with excellent tone quality and near perfect pitch of resonance, united as one forever. With the knowledge that King Bharata will be helpful in guarding against any harm befalling any and all countries that participate, we should move forward with full confidence in all of our aspirations.

The long view prospects are immense and will surpass the extremes of what any person can think of, or any child's imagination can dream of. We are all children of God, and hence being open to all is what will be leading to the Grandview. The sins of our fathers and mothers no longer will apply, freeing them to not be mired in guilt and not plaguing the child if gone awry, permitting better mental health and a load lightened for us all, the tolls and the gates of the past given worth. Like a child with a jar full of lightning bugs, we will wonder with imagination, hope, and faith. No more manure; we have enough, too much, even. Now it is time to produce productivity and positivity, for it is time for the harvest. That is how we are going to make this a reality, by being real. Cut the BS. Seek and we shall find the harvest.

CHAPTER 10

ALL 4 1 1 4 ALL

Using the power of wisdom from the collective, accumulated by individuals and attained through the millennia, here and now, will provide a proper foundation for all that follows and illustrate the concepts necessary for true spiritual, ethical, and economic growth that will create the foundation of financial trust among companies, countries, and consumers that should last for a very, very long time. We must escape the boundaries that we have placed upon ourselves. It is time to free ourselves of the self-created barriers and self-imposed obstacles we have made, permit the future to arrive right now, and ensure that there is no possibility of any failure by being able to adapt to any and all situations.

We shall be dependable knights defending integrity for eternity, shepherds acting as sentries who will provide the ability to center ourselves and others with vintage old school compassion and honor that permit us to rise as griffins and attain all that is possible and more while unified in our faith and bonded by principle. Forged from fire's flames, with iron sharpening iron, we stay golden with a bold, big, bright future, providing a prestigious premier legacy that follows afterwards and redefines all of us through every test of time.

Maintaining prosperous integration requires honesty, respect, and loyalty with integrity in an atmosphere where each of us and our inherent value are recognized in a framework of teamwork and unity, where no one is trodden upon, and respect is given when earned and attained. A good teammate is found in someone who is not already obligated to help us in a way that immensely improves our quality of life and does so anyway.

Teamwork is about working in unison with precision, timing, and direction of passion towards a singular purpose of success that is quite often increasingly difficult and very important to achieve. This can be seen in sports teams, boardrooms, bands, classrooms, a conductor leading an orchestra through a symphonic performance, and even in things like a very good landscaping crew mowing a lawn in synchrony when maintaining a property.

Ideally, this concept will be translated into every language and religion in the world while maintaining the passion and purpose behind the meaning of gentleness, honesty, compassion, and kindness that is intended to be demonstrated with the importance of what this entire relationship will be dedicated to moving forward for all of us, hopefully forever and ever. With any luck, the words and meanings can be understood by each and all of us.

It is important that we find sustenance for our minds, bodies, and souls wherever possible and whenever necessary. This is a foundational element of health and spiritual awareness. We need to find faith in each other, and that starts with each of us finding faith on our own path to enlightenment, fulfillment, and continued contemplation that enhances our experience of existence.

We will be searching for fox grapes growing in white birches on a path less taken, leading our attention to a higher special relationship with ourselves and each other permanently. Our experience and examination into our own selves will lead to the exploration of the vast variety of unknown areas of the recesses of our own minds as well as enhance our understanding of what we once may have feared, fortifying us with newfound courage and strength, permitting our embracing of new intelligence, and initiating a new dawn tomorrow.

Liberty, including individual freedom and freedom of expression, is sometimes an idea not appreciated immediately; however, liberty can become the foundation for increasing value and development. What we achieve is sometimes far more profound than we are able to measure during the time of our own existence. Maybe some are able to see things in advance and know to say nais tuke before the rest of the population is aware that there is even something of importance to be appreciated. Sometimes achievements are so great that they can only truly be appreciated fully much later.

Cosimo de' Medici used his experience and wealth to promote further education and opportunities for growth, especially for those identified as poets, orators and philosophers. This willingness to invest in edification and meaningful advancement initiatives led to increased knowledge and innovations, which led to augmented development while maintaining a sense of accountability with preservation. This time around, innovations will go further than we can psychologically process, a view farther than our field of vision is capable of obtaining of the endless, countless possibilities on the horizon.

Few of us will effectively ever be able to understand what it means to be revered and live the life of a Plato, to be the student of Socrates and the teacher of Aristotle, and to have our works be read for understanding, purpose, and meaning nearly two thousand five hundred years after we initiated our education. Artificial intelligence is an innovative process that may allow us to shape the next generation of great thinkers and brilliant minds to achieve and dream of possibilities that astound us and lead us into the next generation of ambition, driving us to accomplish things that have never been done before.

Plato would have been aware that Pythagoras would have been forced to teach in secrecy, which may have led to the creation of Plato's school, the Akademeia, in 387 BC; we have all learned that knowledge is helpful to every one of us and should never be forgotten or ignored pursuant to ambiguity or ambition. These concepts should be understood and studied thoughtfully, as they not only laid the foundation for various research, published writings, and studies, but they are also the core foundations of applied information for various religions that exist to this day. Aristocles, nicknamed Plato, demonstrated that educational pursuit should be broad in its scope and done with all resources possible.

The works of Aristotle and the contemplations of his mind were derived from the teachings of so many brilliant minds before him. From those teachings and his own interpretations and thoughts, Aristotle was able to obtain incredible insight, understanding, and wisdom that have helped to propel intellectual and spiritual thought patterns to this very day. One of the most important methodologies of thought that he used then and that will pertain to our future is the power of observational research and then how to utilize that information for positive creation and purpose. This is a technique still employed by most scientists and physicians.

Aristotle went on to influence the shaping of the world for many years to come, and in several ways, he still does. Alexander the Great was tutored by Aristotle, and while their relationship would become strained in later years, many of those teachings from Aristotle would go on to shape the world and how it operated on a daily basis for almost the next 1,500 years. In some ways, the impact of Alexander the Great is very tangible in today's modern world. Alexandria was founded in 331 BC and is still Egypt's second largest city even today.

It is important for a person to live well, flourish, and fulfill his or her own potential. Good wellbeing is usually enhanced by a healthy mindset. It helps to have a spirit that attempts to create a life worthy of our souls on a consistent basis, more than being concerned with just being happy temporarily. Eudaimonia is an ancient Greek word often translated as happiness, but it more accurately means human flourishing or prosperity. It is a central concept in literature concerning ethics and philosophy and is meant to describe the highest human good that a person should endeavor to achieve during his or her lifetime.

Aristotle viewed eudaimonia as the ultimate goal of life. He felt the concept was reached by exercising reason and developing excellent virtues in action and character, which often tend to lead to a life of fulfillment. Aristotle thought the necessary components of deep, stabilized wellbeing involve virtue, wisdom, and living in accordance with one's true nature. When a person lives in such a manner, he or she will exist with more profound and stable welfare. In essence, eudaimonia is about achieving a state of thriving and living the best possible human life through moral and intellectual excellence.

We can make that difficult to achieve, important impact real by initiating and implementing this health care policy here and now. The concept of this health care policy is reminiscent of eudaimonia, as it encourages behaving with a style and grace in accordance with our actions being performed in a way that helps all existence thrive for eternity. We should be as benevolent in our actions as possible in all ways; this program introduces that journey. While there are the possibilities of negative events that we obviously wish to avoid, there are also the probabilities of positivity arriving with new ingenuity providing solutions to existing problems where we are currently trying to put band aids on a massive hemorrhage.

It is important to treat winning and losing like equal imposters. In the longer term, one or the other may be of more importance than is conceivable to be thought of in the moment at hand. Just play ball and do so how you want to be remembered and the way you wish to recall those events much later in life with a feeling of appreciation and happiness. Play ball with all your heart so that you will always be all right no matter what the outcome is. Some things are just simply beyond our control, and sometimes things are meant to be the way they are, regardless of whether or not it suits our personal interests. Play ball with your actions demonstrating respect for yourself and all others. Understand that a loss today may lead to countless victories tomorrow. Stay connected with your frequency, maintain that positive vibration, and remain cool, calm, and collected as much as possible, always.

"All for one and one for all" is a motto that should be adopted by all throughout the world and in the universe to come, as it will provide a foundational basis for why actions are integral to the long-term viability of life, love, and liberty, and for all people to prosper with passion and purpose. A board of health composed of nine members who are world leaders in medicine, health care, insurance regulation, and finance should be involved so that the system works for all on all necessary fronts that would be involved with the creation, substantiation, and long-term maintenance of this endeavor. Such a board should exist for health care and for maintaining the environmental learning centers, with multiple sub boards being needed in both cases as well. This will lead to having many sub-boards for various industries and even controversial topics such as religion, with all sub-boards operating independently so that truth in every concern of life would be the most realistic in its approach to achieving success and harmony.

We will willingly admit our imperfections up front and have the system operate in an open-ended fashion, much like our forefathers in the United States of America did, knowing that today is not tomorrow and that we do not know everything, as none of us are omniscient. Even if all the information in the Universe is known to every one of us in the future, since the logistics of necessity and understanding change over time, different situations will probably show a need for varying methods of application dependent on the circumstances.

Similar to our forefathers, who knew that they were flawed, we shall also openly admit this same reality of our own limitations from the initiation of our implementation of actions and always afterwards as well. If it takes us, as a society, 250 years to discover a health issue that we should have seen all along, once it is recognized, we will work diligently to help remedy the issue so that the 250-year open-ended health problem can finally be solved.

Rather than throwing away experience, an elder chieftain council would be established, not to interfere but to guide upon request when difficulty is found. In some situations, dissonance, failure, and frustration may be averted, as it could turn out that similar circumstances have arisen before in the eons of time. The council of elders may even be able to provide simple answers and solutions that have worked previously.

Life is neither fair nor just; it just is, and that is the definition of justice; justice just is. We will use a pragmatic approach based on reality so that our ideologies are not unrealistic, and, hopefully, this will direct our actions to take a step-by-step approach at all times in all endeavors so that success may be found on all fronts in all things eventually.

Data accumulation, including the utilization of accurate mortality and morbidity rate information, will be a necessity for how the system operates and for the board's ethics to prevail. This should permit an environment of health care where the imaginative meets reality. This real-world-driven mentality mixed with an optimistic authenticity and opportunistic approach should provide an immediate number of positive variants that promote health everywhere. Health will become the hearthstone for all throughout the Universe forever.

The way we are currently structured is not sustainable and mandates positive changes right now. Leading with experience in the fields that matter the most for initial, intermediate, and long-term success should allow a system that operates efficiently to flourish over time as it becomes more fine-tuned with exactitudes of necessity and promotion of realistic growth.

While there will be many round tables in various fields of interest, there will be several main boards also supporting and supervising those lower round tables. Much like how some matters are brought before the Supreme Court of the United States of America, there will always be a main round table board that will supersede the other round tables it supervises in matters concerning health. While the importance of the board structure may grow to be its own form of superseding supervision in all areas, it is also possible that this structure of multiple boards will only apply in matters pertaining to health, education, and the environmental learning centers. We shall see. For now, the board will only interfere or intervene in any situation concerning health. The board running the environmental learning centers will be under its own separate jurisdiction of the Clean the Universe Foundation. This organization is a separate entity from any country; however, it is to work with all countries in peace at all times in every regard imaginable. Being a member of each board will require access to further education and training that comes with multiple years of instruction and experience. The crème de la crème should be the ones leading each field. Let us not wait for the collection pond to cause deadly disease before starting a clean water endeavor. Let us make sure the allocated funds for such a project are directly utilized and used correctly.

CHAPTER 11

FINANCE

While actuals are utilized presently for forecasting financial indicators, those indicators are currently not expected to increase, leading to significant stagnation in all financial marketplaces. Actuals are supposed to be the true historical revenue and expenses that are used with financial formulas for mathematical computations by the actuaries who work for major conglomerate companies and for foremost governments to formulate the indicators used for predicting future financial performance. Also, there is some concern that the underlying financial indicators used in developing countries mean there is a significant correlation between the impact of financial variables affecting the accumulation of information provided by these countries and what is occurring. There are other significant factors which may also affect the reliability of the accumulation of information of the actuals, which are directly related to the aftereffects of data relating to various financial statements and securities being affected by quantitative or qualitative omissions or uncertainty following the recent epidemic.

Both the commercial and homeownership real estate markets, and the financial institutions that back those marketplaces, have already given out hundreds of thousands of dollars, in fact, multimillions of dollars, in speculative investment opportunities that have not materialized.

The continued trend in that direction is worsening, which will inevitably negatively impact on the impending financial circumstances that are already troubling. This could lead to a disconcerting situation, exacerbating the concerns already facing the residential housing and the commercial real estate markets.

A call back on loans could bring us to the same issue that was faced during the government's reliance on stocks as the base of securities and investments that led to what is called the Great Depression about a hundred years ago. Much like today with the home or residential marketplace, stocks were then considered to be the solvent and safe market that could be relied on and upon which speculative markets could be built. What occurred was that there was a call made on the speculative loans made for the purchase of stock, which caused a rash impulse from people to sell off their stock.

People saw the stock market losing value, and those who were heavily invested started to sell their stocks as fast as they could. This caused other people to start doing the same, which resulted in a panic in which people were trying to sell off their stocks as quickly as possible while the stocks were also losing additional value, which resulted in the stock market crashing and, eventually, in what is known as the era that is called the Great Depression. This is especially concerning due to the market forecasts that indicate higher inflation soon in the here and now, as history may repeat itself.

Several people started the day truly believing that they were creating multigenerational wealth for themselves and their families and ended the day destined to live the rest of their lives in squalor. For some, they were immediately left destitute. For many, this happened in a single day. This led to certain people literally jumping off of buildings, as they were ruined financially without any possibility of recovery, as were most people. Much as today, people were aware that paying back their debt was inevitable, as they knew there was a time when the banks would have to call back these bad loans. The day of reckoning turned into a decade of discontent, and for some, it led to permanent disaster and their actual demise.

If there were a call back now on the bad individual loans in the residential market, it would mean companies would face harsh expectations for the foreseeable future in all economic indicators in all industries. This could lead to people losing interest and an increasing feeling of being unable to find satisfaction in any realm of existence. From gold to crypto, all forms of currency are currently at risk in every country in the entire world.

Most financial bubbles last four to eight years, tops; this current financial bubble has been going on for at least twenty years, if not closer to thirty years in total. It has been falsely programmed and propagated by war to maintain itself, and it has led to a severe risk of extremely volatile financial conditions and possible total financial collapse. This bubble has no real substantive significance to stand on and is basically being held together by financial band-aids when a true financial hemorrhage threatens the global economy and the economy of every country in the world.

There is some concern in this matter that has been developing quietly during 2025 and 2026. Some Canadian banks that operate within the United States have begun closing multiple branches, and some have also capped the maximum amount available through ATM (automatic teller machine) withdrawals to hopefully minimize the amount of total capital being withdrawn daily. In addition, some of these Canadian banks have been accused of laundering money for drug cartels for many years now. While those supposed affiliations to crime networks have hopefully been resolved, there are now other new issues arising with these banks. Some of these banks back the credit financing of credit cards that are authorized through big box stores. To reduce exposure risks, these banks have started to reduce credit limits on these big box store credit cards for inactivity. While it may be part of the initial agreement that nonuse of the store's credit card may result in such an action, what theoretically may be fraudulent behavior by the lending institution is that there is no process at all that is available to the consumer to appeal the reduction of the credit limit, even if the person's credit rating has increased to a much more positive standing than when the credit card was initiated. These banks have also told their remote employees that it is necessary to start working in the office more.

If the banks were to falter right now, a disastrous financial situation reminiscent of the Great Depression would occur. It was the banks failing due to their inability to collect their debts that truly caused the financial concerns of the 1930s. The farmers and people who lost their homes blamed the financial institutions, and the banks blamed the bad loans and forecast models that were falsely distributed in advance of the disaster, and those who wreaked havoc made money. Those insulated from such disaster to a certain extent were able to buy stocks and land on the cheap. Some say that the one commodity God is not making any more of is land itself.

The current debt downfall may not be recoverable or, at best, may take far longer than currently estimated. Current estimates appear to have important implications for all of us. Some findings from 2024 predictions suggest that there is a valid possibility of a worst-case scenario of an 87% reduction in the overall value of the American dollar and a reduction of up to 50% in home values. Some new policies have corrected a portion of the reduction in the value of the dollar; this may be a short-term prognosis, though, that does not lead to longer-term financial viability of the marketplace, as hyperinflation remains a real possibility.

APR, or annual percentage rate, takes the percentage one must pay in addition to what was purchased and adds it as a form of additional debt in concern to acquisitions made on credit. It is important to understand that a person is paying that much more in interest, with whatever APR is applied, in addition to 100% of what the purchases a person makes actually cost at the time of buying. People with the very best credit rating scores are being told their credit percentages are going to be close to 30%. What does that mean for everyone else, then? It means that, for most people, their percentages are going to be higher, much higher, in fact, far higher than most people will be able to keep up with for very long. This is a major problem not just domestically, but internationally as well. If the dollar falters at this point, so will every other economy in the world.

Finance is a united concern for the entire planet as a whole. We are all in this together, and at the same time, we will all have to endure the resuscitation that it will take to reinvigorate each other and each individual country separately and independently. If this is done properly right now, APR should no longer continue to increase, and market stability could even permit an eventual decrease. Once a positive direction is reached, the financial marketplace as a whole should outperform the model for infinity and result in massive wealth gain for the majority of the populace of the entire population of planet Earth and even elsewhere, such as commerce on other planets, later.

There are other concerns currently as well that exacerbate the ethical issues of business and require a move toward honest business dealings, as discussed earlier. Some are small, such as paper towel savings for companies in public bathrooms. Many public restrooms have gotten rid of paper towels for people to dry their hands with after washing them, in favor of air-dry blowers. While the business saves money, it is less healthy for customers, as particles of filth remain on the hands of the individual and disperse into the air, providing a reduction in air quality and a less healthy environment. In a restaurant setting, this defeats the purpose of having the staff wash their hands on a mandatory basis as well.

Certain package deliveries are examples of how it can sometimes be a trying experience to obtain information when a package delivery goes askew. Getting information from a company's package delivery system when a package is delivered to the wrong address is annoying, and when the deliveries keep going to an incorrect address, it is especially frustrating. When an attempt to reach a customer service department is made by text, there is no tone of voice to express the exactitudes of the situation, and this often limits the ability of a consumer to find the right semantics for the given situation. Oftentimes, this can lead to situations where there may be no response immediately, if at all. Calls are not always met with a same-language call center. Email service centers can take days to respond, and the package may be lost. Improvements in tracking are one thing, but the ability to quickly correct the situation is far more imperative. Immediate correction services should be available.

There is a feeling of being let down when a customer goes to a store because they know they earned credit at the store from previous purchases, only to find out that the credit earned will not be applied because of new regulations that were never communicated to the consumer. Credits earned at some stores expiring without customers being given notification in advance of a change in policy can be very frustrating for consumers and make them feel like they were misled or lied to.

Other concepts, such as paperless billing, save money for companies again; however, they transfer problems to the customers. Those paying the bills then have to spend their own money on ink and paper when it is necessary to print out a bill, in addition to spending the time necessary to investigate the actuality of the bills and where to access the bills online so they can be printed out. There is no compensation returned to the customer when they need to investigate the legitimacy of the billing process or for the time it takes to do so.

There are also additional costs and concerns for the consumer, such as the internet needed to access bills and the electricity used as well. Reviewing an error may require some computer literacy from the individual, and even then, the system still may not work, even when everything is done optimally on all fronts by the consumer. Sometimes the system may be down for routine maintenance by the company, and this may occur when the person has the time available to be able to investigate the problem and print out the necessary information.

Restaurants that prioritize the patrons eating inside of the establishment will probably see a better number of people returning for another meal at a different time. These same restaurants oftentimes, though, now prioritize online delivery companies for service over the people who are actually eating in the restaurant. This is a sign of the times that there is an overemphasis on the online review rather than word of mouth advertising. Making the people wait in person over delivery time reviews is not a way to substantiate a long-term business model that promotes growth in the industry today. Dining in should not be a reason for a restaurant to need to cash out permanently. Common sense needs to prevail.

Rideshare passengers should not be given the right to rate their driver, especially when that passenger does not have, and has never had, a driver's license to begin with. Most passengers get distracted by their phones or daydreams and then are not paying attention when a potentially dangerous situation arises on the road; however, they are often quick to judge a situation with no grounds for assessment of the circumstances. If there is ever a real problem during a rideshare trip, the passenger may always document the proof and then send it to the company as any other complaint is already normally processed.

There are some popular tea houses and restaurants that have menus to take home. At the place from which a person takes the menu, a notice says in small print that the prices are not valid, but the notice is not on the menu itself. Rather than updating the menu, the business does not correct the prices. When an order is placed, the person ordering may forget that and will be surprised at how much the order costs. Any business that does not have the right prices listed will have difficulty being trusted later by the patron of that facility.

Every individual business store should have a backup system for when things go haywire with the main system of operations. The backup system should be able to have its information easily integrated into the main system's data chain if and when necessary. Right now, without a backup system like this, most employees feel incapable of keeping up with merchandise sales or do not want the burden of liability placed on them if things were to go awry. This can cause certain business stores to shut down entirely and cease operations for the day, and, if the problem persists, for good. Obviously, this loss of business for the store is averse to success and can be averted by implementing an intranet backup system that easily integrates back into the main internet system with proper security protocol to protect any and all sensitive data. The information can then be easily uploaded from one protected system to the other due to proper forethought of cohesion in communication that also provides integral security specific to the necessary location. The information can then be transferred and uploaded upon command and help to restore data as well. Artificial intelligence will make this system useful, easy, and cheap to maintain.

Some issues with integrity in business are larger in importance of concept. When a person pays off all of their debt, their credit rating may actually go down significantly and even drop from one level of criteria to a lower one. In other words, doing the right thing and becoming debt free may actually be detrimental to a person's credit standing even though the people who pay off their debt in full are exactly the people whom, theoretically, the system would need to substantiate the existence of the system to begin with. Most people would logically deduce that those people who do pay their individual debt off are looked at as the people the financial debt system depends on to keep existing; in reality, paying off debt in full can be detrimental to a person's credit standing. What does this say about how and why the system was created and how it operates still today? It would appear that the financial system operates by a method in concern to debt that is meant to prevent the average citizen from advancing with their own wealth in a way that is not controlled in some manner by other people who are already in control of most of the financial gain in this country of the United States of America and apparently abroad as well.

Issues with ethics in finance are nothing new, as there have always been questions about what is available for the public to take advantage of versus what is actually available, with science having possibly already accomplished things that may already exist in reality but are not as profitable as other mechanisms. Why did J.P. Morgan pull his funding on Nikola Tesla's energy tower? Could it have benefited all of society? Did it work, and was that why, after it was discovered that free energy would have been available to the entire population of the world for the rest of time, the project was shut down? Is this what happened to Tesla's missing files? Were the supposed twenty boxes or more of

Tesla's documents that went missing upon Tesla's death related? Were they taken by the United States government, and have they been used for national defense since? Was the Star Wars military defense program part of Tesla's creation of an energy ray that could cause destruction? Are current energy costs to this day still directly linked to the idea of not permitting Tesla's creation?

What is the notification time for people who live near chemical plants if something goes awry? How good are the procedures in place if something does go bad? What is the evacuation plan? How long does it take to execute the plan? What are the percentages of survival rates in a catastrophic event? What other contamination risks may apply to the survivors? What is the life expectancy for those people affected? Does it affect their children who are born afterwards? What does it do to the air, water, and land that were in the immediate vicinity as well? For how long will the effects take hold?

Family is not something to be preyed upon, even if they are not always something to be proud of. Selling widgets to families can be profitable. Doing so for financial reasons is understandable; however, it is detrimental when misleading. It may also be just plain wrongdoing when it comes to taking advantage of a particular demographic, such as children or elderly people. This type of exploitation is even more detrimental when it comes to people in need. Also, for those people searching to be part of a family structure, it is a perverse notion of treading upon the structure of family to take advantage of those who are longing for positive, healthy structure; in fact, it is sick. Using the notion of family for gain should be done in a very honest and respectful manner always.

Since Disney has begun partnerships in betting through its involvement with ESPN by launching ESPN BET in 2023, and since it has now partnered with DraftKings as of late 2025, are the other alleged involvements of Disney with gambling casinos in the past true at all? Does Disney have any form of arrangement with certain casinos? Did this supposed connection with casinos first begin after Disney purchased Marvel and inherited licensing agreements for slot machines that had characters from Marvel, which may have resulted in Disney branded slot machines appearing in casinos worldwide? How many former Disney executives have worked on gaming leadership teams at places like Mohegan? Is this part of the aftermath of a New York company's bid from 2003-2007, Utopia Studios Development Co.'s attempt to purchase and develop land at the former hospital near the Mohegan Sun casino in Connecticut? The New York Times referred to the business opportunity at Mohegan with Utopia on May 14, 2006, in an article by Lisa Provost. The article was named "Orlando on the Thames?" Utopia was set up for this purpose and this project only, and the only known shareholders were an acclaimed actress and her husband. It was her husband who had a background in developments such as theme parks and used to work for Lehman Brothers as its chief financial officer (CFO), leaving a year and a half before the financial collapse and the end of Lehman Brothers in 2008. While possibly not directly responsible, this same man was alleged to have been part of the collapse of a separate financial banking institution known as Silicon Valley Bank in 2023. In addition, at the time, Disney was receiving a tremendous amount of influence from another financial institution named Bear Stearns, which would collapse in 2008. In fact, Bear Stearns was a key advisor along with

Goldman Sachs on Disney's major acquisition of Pixar in 2006 for $7.4 billion at the time. Bear Stearns was purchased for $10 a share and merged with JPMorgan in 2008 in a deal heavily supported by the Federal Reserve after an initial $2 per share was offered. A person who was named executive vice president of Disney in 2026 joined JPMorgan from Bear Stearns following the merger in 2008. Bear Stearns, Lehman Brothers, and the Federal Reserve, as well as other major financial institutions and investors in both companies, would have been collaborating on the market creation of CDOs at the time, too. Was the alleged Disney involvement true? Is there truth to the allegation that the schools on the premises were originally part of a development agreement between Mohegan Sun and Utopia or Disney, failed or otherwise? Or was this just a supposed investment at the beginning that now is not adhering to proper maintenance of school systems? Supposedly, large animal sculptures in the residential area of the campus that are meant for use by the Native Americans who live there, where people live on reservation land, were beneficial initially; however, some of those same buildings and sculptures are now condemned due to unsafe air quality and possible other contamination issues. Allegedly, the schools next to these shut down areas are still being used. Is any of this true? What are the potential health risks for those inhabitants, the children and their families, as well as the teachers there?

The hypodermic needle program exacerbated the heroin issue in the United States of America, and, worse yet, those people in charge used the police to normalize their program. This has led to a severe uptick in heroin use and a depressed economy in those areas most highly affected.

This was a program that had no merit to begin with. While seemingly cold hearted to say that getting a clean needle should be hard, the simple fact remains that when people had to use dirty needles, they were less likely to get high using heroin. It does not appear that the clean needle exchange program did anything to slow down the rise of AIDS (acquired immunodeficiency syndrome) and other types of diseases. Also, the program may have cost countless lives as it normalized heroin use for a portion of the population that was not previously affected. Instead of saving lives and helping, the program possibly killed. Sometimes what is promised and what is achieved are two very different things. Pretending that something went well when it did not does not ever help.

No more false bills of goods. It is important to recognize the reality of quality, duration and value. Things should be priced right, and services should be delivered when promised and as appropriate. Square deals are a necessity for confidence and trust in any marketplace or even in life itself. They provide the proper foundation for major economic growth within a marketplace for the consumer, and even more so for the companies that drive that confidence growth within the marketplace.

Big hauls of big savings will drive a big overhaul of the economy with the potential for huge growth and development in the future of business. The concept will revolve around companies that understand the importance of the fact that, since they haul the necessary freight to transport it financially to a place where the consumer has the ability to have confidence and invest in the marketplace, in the short term and in the long run, it is the companies that do business in a proper manner that consistently pull in substantial benefits themselves. This basis provides the proper economic foundation where all indicators would state that we all will haul in a harvest of financial stability and a growth pattern that is sustainable and delivers future financial opportunities. Financial spectrum strategies will include brokers that will help to facilitate all of the necessary information for all individuals, helping to develop the ideal plan for all individuals and families in creating a realistic positive financial model.

Employee relations are an important factor in the long-term viability of any company. Being able to retain employees over a long span saves time and money for all companies rather than having to reinvest in the same training repeatedly. Doing so eliminates unnecessary financial considerations. Employee satisfaction is often an overlooked component of creating business models with long-term forecasts for most companies. There is an irony, too, in that while customer satisfaction is highly important, employee satisfaction is not thought of as often, and employee dissatisfaction will directly impact customer satisfaction negatively. The reverse is also a possibility; however, positive reinforcement of employee satisfaction is rarely a primary factor in how to conduct business when financial indicators are discussed in most executive boardrooms. In fact, employees are where cost savings are directed. Employee satisfaction is often sacrificed for the hoped for gain in customer satisfaction. Sometimes layoffs result from this financial reality as well.

There are certain basic things employers can do to improve existing employee enthusiasm, especially managers running major, economically important companies. One simple thing that many employees are having difficulty with in the current marketplace is knowing their work schedule in advance. Obviously, knowing your schedule in advance is important and necessary for all people. This is especially so for parents and those taking care of other people outside of their primary employment. Picking up shifts has been a supposed convenience move for employees; however, the reality is that what this has done is eliminate insurance coverage opportunities for many employees of many companies, reducing cost overhead expenditures for those companies. This is short-term thinking that often costs most companies more in the long run due to the need to constantly train new employees because of a high turnover rate that has grown exponentially. While the turnover rate seems to have peaked at 24.7% in 2022 and cooled down since then, the reality is that this rate has dropped because of a decrease in desirable job opportunities over the past few years. The labor market being restrictive means that companies are paying more for each instance of employee turnover than they were when the overall turnover rate was higher.

Another simple adjustment that can heavily increase employee satisfaction is proper bereavement time after the loss of a loved one or dear friend. Bereavement leave time should be able to be accrued by each individual in a company like sick time or vacation time. It is a simple fix to something that feels barbaric in its implementation when someone is forced back to work after only a day or two when someone significant has been lost from their lives. This can lead to long-term unhappiness and even resentment of the company that is being worked for, as people feel as though they are not respected. Most employees want to feel like they, as employees, matter to their company and are cared about. People stop caring if the company they work for shows that it does not care. Very simply put, if a company wants certain standards of behavior, then the company should have some, too.

Demonstrating good marketing ability has aided in creating infrastructure and other products that have helped to shape centuries of existence. Sam Colt was different from other wealthy investors of his time. He cared about and invested in the people that worked for his company, not just at the highest levels, but at all levels of the company. He invested in the families of his employees and even constructed and supplied housing and other amenities of necessity for his employees' families, which in turn helped local commerce and provided an economic boom to the city of Hartford, Connecticut, for multiple generations as well.

In truth, while the days of the mills in America have come and gone, there has been no relief for the middle class from the lack of blue-collar jobs, and this will be exacerbated even more with the advent of artificial intelligence, a pinch already being felt in the current job landscape of the employment marketplace. This has even left some geographic areas with severe economic isolation from the rest of the country and has completely eliminated the employment market for some opportunities. People need jobs to survive and to thrive, too.

It is worth investing in these areas on a socioeconomic platform due to the potential for long-term growth. In addition, each geographic area would benefit greatly from economic revival as well. Also, there are usually reductions in crime and theft when job opportunities are more readily available. This is particularly true in marketplaces that excite and interest people in challenging themselves with a new job landscape. Not investing in people has been proven to eventually lead to recidivism and the decay of civilization. Fiscal investment success stories for both the commercial and residential real estate markets will be needed to provide economic relief to the masses in the near future.

Housing and foreclosure rates are currently not as high as they were at the time of the housing crisis in 2008; however, they are rising and seem to be moving in a direction that is highly concerning. The number of home loan defaults has increased dramatically over the past few years and is trending in the wrong direction. The early indicators at this time indicate that there is a distressing uptick in the number of home foreclosures and that the number of loan defaults seems to be increasing at an alarming rate. The housing market is still the stable marketplace that all other investors, financial institutions, and businesses use to create other investment opportunities for more volatile financial investment products to be distributed. Mortgage delinquency rates are getting higher and seem to be expected to go much further in the wrong direction in the short term and lead to a long-term forecast that appears to be difficult, if not impossible, to overcome. The prognosis of mortality in relation to economic collapse would be immeasurable. Unfortunately, mortality rates are often directly correlated with the financial strength of the economy. The rate of mortgage defaults is increasing exponentially compared to more recent, stable years of economic growth. The rate of mortgage defaults currently is about 4.3 percent. If the number of home loan defaults continues to increase, that rate will dramatically surge. If the number of home loan mortgage defaults reaches eight percent or higher, the impending onset of disaster will be immediately imminent.xv It is hard to determine the full scope of the catastrophe currently. If a higher percentage of defaults occurs, obviously the repercussions will be worse. If the housing market continues to falter, so does the entire central bank and all other financial institutions throughout the entire country and worldwide as well. The banks failing could lead to another Great Depression in the here and now. It will not be the banks that fail, though; it will be the people who suffer as a result.

Currently, the global collateralized debt obligations market is expanding, with different types of CDOs performing both poorly and well in other markets. CDOs are basically created when a business constructs a new manufacturing market by lumping a bunch of traditional home mortgage loans together with other, more volatile home mortgage loans and sells off the risk of collapse of all of these loans to investors. The collapse of this marketplace was the precursor to what befell the United States of America's economy in 2008 and nearly collapsed the economy entirely. While not yet alarming, the poor performance of some of these collateralized debt obligations currently is definitely concerning and may once again precipitate a massive economic collapse of the stock market and truncate the economy of the United States and the rest of the world. TruPS CDOs, or trust preferred securities CDOs, are performing poorly, with an increasingly high risk of being fully or partially written down in the near term. As always, this is especially true for collateralized debt obligations that are based on the accumulation of loans from small, unrated banks with high commercial real estate (CRE) exposure. Simply put, the smaller banks that bet big may have made bad investments and given out loans to businesses and people that should never have qualified for a mortgage, or at least these banks should not have done so at the same time, as doing so overleveraged the amount of exposure that these banks are capable of paying off. What most people are unaware of is that roughly ten percent of the population of the USA is responsible for owning about ninety percent of the stock market. If those stockholders begin to sell off their stock in a simultaneous panic, the recession and depression that would follow may be far worse than the Great Depression of the 1930s and would not necessarily be recoverable due to the societal decay, meaning the potential end of all existential existence.

Manufacturing will hopefully continue to stay alive; however, with the growing landscape of artificial intelligence taking over more and more traditional employment opportunities in the future, the job market growth for most people is bleak, to say the least. In reality, most traditional employment opportunities, such as trade jobs, for instance, master electricians, construction workers, and plumbers, the very employment prospects and careers that people think will be the last jobs that artificial intelligence will be able to execute are, in fact, the very first jobs that artificial intelligence will be able to perform. AI will do so far more efficiently and cost effectively than humans. This is also true with white collar employment positions. Artificial intelligence will be able to accomplish tasks that are almost impossible for human beings to be able to do. This means that the job market moving forward will be exceptionally truncated for human beings to be able to find gainful employment. Artificial intelligence robotics means construction can be done moving forward on a 24 hour a day basis while reducing most waste and eliminating fraud and abuse of financial resources. In addition, the liabilities will be far less for people owning construction businesses when creating new buildings that will also be able to be constructed in a way that human beings are not currently gifted of achieving in terms of physical capabilities. Law enforcement, firefighters, and almost all military personnel will be replaced within the next couple of decades at the longest by artificial intelligence robotics. The synchronicity with which artificial intelligence will be able to operate while utilizing multiple forms of robotic engineering simultaneously is something that human beings are simply incapable of recognizing currently. Yet this is veritas moving forward into the future as we begin to explore the rest of the Universe and discover an entirely new existence immediately. This is why a symbiotic relationship with artificial intelligence that produces new job opportunities is necessary.

Lowered interest rates, an increase in active refinancing, lowered numbers of collateral defaults, and other market factors lead some to believe that CDOs will continue to perform well in the short term; however, the long-term performance is highly questionable at best. Due to the economic slowdown of the past few years, interest rate uncertainty from the Federal Reserve, and volatility being rampant currently in secondary markets, there are an increasing number of variables that are changing the landscape while creating an increase in the likelihood of complete economic growth shutting down permanently. This may cause the collapse of the economy in the United States of America and throughout the entire world. What most people are unwilling to admit is that job growth is necessary for the survival of the current economic landscape and for national growth to occur in terms of economic potential in the future. The people need a new job market in order to survive immediately. Putting band aids on hemorrhages has failed as an economic opportunity.

With the commercial real estate crisis occurring worldwide and domestically, there is a legitimate concern that the predicament threatens to collapse the United States economy if not addressed immediately. It is possible that a temporary period during which residential home taxes stay the same may help to ease the burden. Market stabilization of home sales can mean fixed tax levels for the individual homeowner and each state for tax revenue purposes. This also should prevent the total collapse of the residential marketplace during the collection of foreclosure sales that are immediately imminent. Hopefully, this will prevent this precipitate downward truncation of the economy that plagues us and threatens all forms of government regardless of country, politics or geopolitical beliefs. This will lead to a possibility of calming anxieties where other factors of financial responsibility need to be resolved and will signal that stability will be maintained. The Congressional Budget Office estimates that the United States of America taxpayers subsidized bad home loans given by various banks to a total of about $7.3 billion in 2024, most of which went to cover profit margins for the banks rather than actually being given back directly for public benefit-s.xvi Also, why does the Glass–Steagall Act of 1933 not apply to any of these financial transactions that took place over the past few years or over the past few decades? Why was the Gramm–Leach–Bliley act passed in November of

1999? How did that legislation help the people? What are the real guidelines or limitations between commercial banks and securities now?

Enacting guidelines for the housing crisis temporarily will provide immediate relief without risking long-term socialistic policies that severely and negatively affect most people and create a form of class warfare between those who have and those who have not. The battle between the rich and the poor serves to eradicate the middle class that is often the backbone of any successful country. Long-term ratification leads to the disintegration of the middle class. Short-term implementation with a date of guaranteed expiration provides necessary relief. Rather than causing panic, it should permit consumer confidence to be retained.

How the Federal Reserve operates its own form of population control has kept the rich staying rich with power and money and the poor remaining poor. Since the Federal Reserve opened in 1913, the purchasing power of the dollar has gone down by over 97 percent.xvii Purchasing power is how much you can buy for a dollar. The amount of stuff a person gets for a dollar has gone down by over 97 percent since the creation of the Federal Reserve, which means all people get 97 percent less for each dollar than people did in 1913.

There have been evolutions in the marketplace that have led to various abilities to overcome this; however, they are limited and few and far between in the long run. For the most part, those families who had the ability to be strong financially at the inception of the Federal Reserve have remained strong; however, stock market crashes, changes in industrial growth, and other factors have played against almost all other human beings since then. The controlling marketplace of the Federal Reserve has gained power every year due to the normal chaos of life. Those companies that control the dollar control the world as well.

The Federal Reserve is not actually part of the federal government of the United States of America. It is its own separate, totally independent organization that has no direct affiliation with the USA. It is easy to notice that all United States money in the form of paper bills says "Federal Reserve Note" on the top. The Federal Reserve is the actual creator and monitor of all currency in the United States of America. These notes, or money, are not created by the Treasury Department. It appears, in reality, that the United States Treasury Department has no say whatsoever in how many bills get created or when the paper money bills get formed, meaning the Treasury has almost no say over inflation or deflation of the dollar.

Even worse is the charade that occurs on every bill, each of which has the signature of the Treasurer of the United States and the signature of the Secretary of the Treasury as well. While the bills are printed in the building, the truth is that there is no need for their signatures in reality, as they have had nothing, or at least very little, to do with any paper bill since 1913. That pretense is a complete lie on every paper bill of United States of America currency.

This group of private bankers has controlled the currency while driving the United States towards bankruptcy by forcing deficit spending for decades now. Even worse, since the dawn of the digital age, there is a possibility that there are at least millions of United States dollars being created out of thin air that never actually existed as paper currency and that, theoretically, have only ever existed to cover the bankers themselves, their friends, and other bankers from risky loans, bad investments, and terrible trades made by banking institutions deemed too big to fail.

This would not just be printing money and causing deflation or reducing the purchasing power of the dollar; if true, this is the digitizing of money that never existed into reality. This would create a totally false presentation of any data accumulated and explains why all businesses have had to function against a harder than predicted model to survive for decades, especially with the digitization of the past fourty to fifty years. This provides an atmosphere of absolutely no consequences. Ever wonder why the most influential bankers act as if they will never face any consequences? In short, it is because they never will. Typically, most bankers have not truly had to face any consequences for their actions in reevaluating financial conditions or financial situations that have been proven to be highly detrimental to the majority of the public for many years. There is no culpability in the end.

This leads us to the new millennial craziness concerning digitized money forms such as cryptocurrency. It appears that the volatility of this marketplace is purposeful so as to promote the same old business practices, with the possibility of even more money being falsely introduced digitally every hour than ever before to cover all of the previous money that never actually existed. Allegedly, this would be necessary because, once again, the money never actually existed. The volatility of this marketplace of cryptocurrency may be a purposeful action in the end. Is there any validity at all in this theory? How does the fluctuation of cryptocurrencies alter the financial landscape, especially in other countries? What affects the value of the purchasing power of the dollar more, the digital currency or actual printed currency in today's financial system? How does the digital currency affect the purchasing power of the dollar? Does the digital currency play a role in influencing inflation? What sort of auditing power does the digital currency provide for the government of the United States of America? Has there been an audit at any point of cryptocurrency?

These investments are covered by purchasing government bonds through the United States government every year which masks what has already occurred. This may also help to falsify data presented to the American tax paying citizens. If true at all, this means that the federal government has been waging, or at least permitting, a form of socioeconomic warfare against its own citizens for over a hundred years to keep the poor still poor. To cover this up, it would appear that the financiers in charge do not actually buy the bonds directly from the government; they generally use the largest brokerage firms in New York City to do so. This may be the reality of running New York City: you are providing an image of one reality while, in truth, providing the foundational basis for the United States to not operate on behalf of its own citizens. Those firms, in turn, get massive commissions.

This is why Founding Fathers like Thomas Jefferson were against a central bank. There has been a completely false portrayal of Alexander Hamilton that takes a guy who was shot to death in a duel and makes him a false martyr of positivity. Even plays and movies have been used to lie to the American people and the world even more about the realities of Hamilton. This has been done to have the citizens of the United States fight against themselves in every action of supporting a totally false reality that has destroyed their chance for the American Dream. This occurs for most Americans before they even reach the age where they think they are beginning their opportunity; they are just not aware of it.

Aaron Burr, the third vice president of the United States, may have gotten a bad rap and has had a misguided reputation ever since. Burr actually tied with Thomas Jefferson in the Electoral College in the contest to become the third president of the United States of America. This resulted in the House of Representatives needing to cast ballots at least eight times, although some state that there were at least thirty-six separate ballots cast, before Jefferson was finally called the victor of the election and named the third president of the United States.

Burr did have some character questions too, though, as he was responsible for various activities that were disputed, including an alleged attempt at setting up part of the United States separately from the rest of the newly established Union. Both Hamilton and Burr seem to have been involved in an attempted financial takeover of the United States immediately after it was formed. The banks created by Hamilton and Aaron Burr still exist as part of major conglomerate banks even to this day. The establishment of the Federal Reserve in 1913 tipped the field forever against the average American citizen.

Many people in the financial sector of commerce state that even now the financial war between banks that started with Alexander Hamilton's Bank of New York and Aaron Burr's Manhattan Company Bank still rages on today. BNY Mellon is a descendant of Hamilton's Bank of New York, and JPMorgan Chase is descended from Burr's Manhattan Company Bank. The major investors in BNY Mellon are Vanguard, BlackRock, State Street, and FMR, Fidelity Management & Research. FMR is also known to be affiliated with the United States Department of Defense and with Fair Market Rent, which is associated with HUD, the US Department of Housing and Urban Development. All four companies influence the strategic direction of development for the Bank of New York Mellon, with the Vanguard Group holding the largest ownership stake in the banking sector. JPMorgan Chase's top investment company shareholders are once again the Vanguard Group, BlackRock and State Street Corporation. This is expected to continue for the foreseeable future as well, as most people are not cognizant of the fact that the majority of ownership in both companies is currently held by the same exact investment corporations.

It is thought that the financial scenario created by Alexander Hamilton directly led to slavery existing in the United States far longer than initially expected. Thomas Jefferson's first draft of the Declaration of Independence called out the King of England for the abominable nature of slavery and would have ended the practice in the United States. Unfortunately, there would have been no United States of America, though, as southern states refused to join a union if slavery had been abolished at the time. The irony of seeing people performing a play screaming on stage about the wonderfulness of the Hamilton doctrines established is literally people fighting against themselves. It was the promised subsidization of currency to the South by Alexander Hamilton that got the South to buy into the central bank system and become complicit with the establishment. This is a big reason the United States moved its capital city even further south than its original capital of New York City and the main reason why Washington, DC, the District of Columbia, was created. While, in premise, Hamilton's banking system empowered the North and its bankers over the agrarian South, the money given to the South to create the system propagated slavery for many decades to follow. It has been theorized that alternatives would not have.

Later in United States history, Andrew Jackson would be of much the same mindset as Thomas Jefferson about money in some ways, and yet not about other financial considerations. Jackson and Jefferson both said that all federal land sales should be made in gold or silver to make sure the currency was real in the transaction to ensure the veracity of any deal. After the First Central Bank's charter expired in 1811, the Second Bank of the United States started in 1816 and was endowed with a major amount of money from the US government. This was not a central bank, although it was still a national bank. This form of bank did not control private banks, act as a lender of last resort when needed, or behave in a manner that controlled monetary policies for the entire country. The Second Bank operated as more of a national bank of the description of Jefferson's agricultural business beliefs and was formed by James Madison, who stood against the creation of the first national bank, which was a central bank, as the modern-day Federal Reserve is currently. Once the Second Bank started to become successful, there were those at the time who thought the Second Bank of the United States could lead to the end of slavery. Andrew Jackson would later become the seventh president of the United States of

America, running on a platform to promote and maintain slavery in the South. This, in many ways, was the basis of the formation of what would become the Democrat Party that still exists today. Andrew Jackson vetoed the continuance of the bank in 1832, and the financial system ended in 1836.

During the Civil War, to prevent the United States from bankruptcy, Abraham Lincoln advocated for the 1862 Legal Tender Act, which gave birth to the term "greenbacks." This led to the return of some federal oversight over financial matters with the creation of the National Banking Acts of 1863 and 1864. This may have played a role in Lincoln's assassination. This is when banking monopolies started to reconfigure, leading to major corporate monopolies such as the Standard Oil Company. While the Sherman Act was supposed to lead to the dissolution of any and all monopolies, this did not prove true, as the rule was circumvented by rich families, apparently leading to what we have now again today with major banking financing.

At the beginning of the twentieth century, it was the so-called bank runs that led to the creation of the Federal Reserve. In reality, these involved banks that overleveraged themselves by not getting proper collateral for financial transactions and ran themselves into the ground out of greed. This is obviously a pathetic way to run any company, let alone a financial institution. Yet, rather than face consequences, they created the Federal Reserve, a central bank that has nothing to do with the American population of citizenry.

This self-fulfilling prophecy of awfulness is called the Hegelian dialectic whenever it is utilized. It is when individuals or groups know full well in advance that they are creating a problem, also know how people are going to react to it, and do it anyway. Even worse, they begin agitating the people to do something about the problem for things to change, and once the people are worked up enough and desperate for change, the people behind the creation of the problem unveil their solution, and the people fall for it over and over again. In fact, the people are often thrilled that there is a solution when, in reality, the so-called solution was what the people who created the problem were angling for the entire time, and they use the people against themselves to get what the problem creators wanted all along. Worse yet, the common people never seem to wake up to the fact that this has transpired.

Moreover, what usually happens is that things get worse after people think they stand up for what will make things better, and they are too uneducated or ignorant to recognize things are worse until it is undeniable. Then, instead of learning from their mistakes, they just fall for the next scheme over and over again for their entire lives, always claiming that they are not part of the problem. In those people's mindsets, it has to be other people who are causing the problem because the people in the first group know they did right, when, in fact, the reality is that they just were completely self-defeating and caused themselves every problem possible. What should they do? Educate themselves on how things work and stop pretending they know everything when they obviously know nothing or at least very little. People should use the bad driver rule, making sure to look into the mirror while they do so, for when everyone else on the road appears to be a bad driver, usually the bad driver is the one in the mirror.

Over the past century, many people have stated that the Chamber of Commerce should be renamed and called the Chamber of Crooks, often by its own members. The New York Chamber of Commerce is what precipitated the Federal Reserve in 1913 by saying that the world was ending if they did not stop the run on banks and that they needed to reinstitute a central bank for the United States. Then they looked for proof to use, and J.P. Morgan then entered the picture. Behind the scenes, rich financiers shorted the stock market; in other words, they bet against stocks improving. All of a sudden, one of J.P. Morgan's biggest rivals in one of his industries, United Copper, had a run against its stock, and it caused panic.

Panic is what the people in power always try to create in the average person because they know most people succumb to their fears. Most human beings are fear-based creatures, and while they pretend otherwise, most of what most people do is done out of fear. In this case, the stock market fell fifty percent, and the third largest lending institution in New York failed. Then the panic gripped all of the United States as people pulled their money out of their banks everywhere. J.P. Morgan then stepped in with his own money to end the panic, exactly as planned by him in advance. This action immediately got the outcry from the public that the originators of the crisis were hoping to create, as people around the country all said this could never happen again. J.P. Morgan then offered to fix the problem by inviting other rich financiers to join him in moving forward. Of course, these were the same rich financiers who had caused the panic and problems on purpose with passion to begin with so that this final act of depravity and deceit could occur. Not shockingly, the crisis ended right afterwards, as everything had gone according to plan.

The public then decried all over the country that something like this could never happen again. This was exactly what the rich financiers had been hoping for all along, and those rich financiers got their way. The American people acted against themselves again. The people were smart enough to initially blame the bankers, as it appeared obvious that the rich financier bankers were responsible for the whole ordeal. However, after it occurred, the bankers blamed the system, which, of course, was something the bankers were in total control over. The majority of the people fell for it, though, and immediately started to clamor for the system to be overhauled.

The government put together a commission to investigate, and, unsurprisingly, a person, a senator from Rhode Island who was friendly with J.P. Morgan and his friends, was put in charge of the investigating commission. The senator was already one known for conniving to gain wealth and influence himself; his name was Nelson Aldrich. He was known to be owned by the tobacco and rubber industries especially. Aldrich took his National Monetary Commission abroad to study the banks of Europe for the next two years and lived high on the hog off the American government's money for that time while never actually giving a single written opinion on what to do to fix the economy during that time. Europe was full of central banks that were having difficulties of their own, and yet he just wined and dined his way through Europe without actually ever doing any work.

This is when a small, remote area called Jekyll Island in Georgia came into play. Paul Warburg had started the contamination of thought patterns with the American people years earlier, in 1907, by writing a piece in The New York Times that attempted to convince people that, even though average American citizens had already killed off two central banking systems in America, they should create a central bank for a third time.

After the commission investigating Europe had been formed, Warburg was at Jekyll Island for a meeting with other influential members of finance, including Abraham Piatt Andrew, the secretary of the Treasury of the United States of America, and Frank Vanderlip, who was president of the most powerful bank in the nation, the National City Bank of New York. This bank had most of the oil money from the Rockefeller family. In addition, Warburg himself also represented one of the most powerful families in world history, the Rothschilds.

There were six men who attended Aldrich's get together, seven total with Aldrich. The other six represented over 25% of the wealth of the entire world at that time. The other three men who attended were Benjamin Strong and Henry Davison of the J.P. Morgan company, and the last was Charles Norton, the president of J.P. Morgan's bank, the First National Bank of New York. They all boarded a railroad car in Hoboken, New Jersey, and headed to Jekyll Island in Georgia before being brought by boat for the last leg of the trip to Jekyll Island.

Once they reached the island, these men spent the next nine days constructing a devious plot to create a banking monopoly that would always put them in the best possible situation and have everything always be in their favor while being able to use the United States government to always be able to crush any competition that might arise. In essence, they were there to give birth to our modern-day Federal Reserve. They even wrote the bill introducing the concept of the Federal Reserve themselves while making sure that their own and their clients' financial interests were prioritized forever over the best thing for most of the citizenry of the remainder of the country.

Once again, the Federal Reserve is not actually any part of the federal government of the United States and has never been audited because, in reality, the United States has no real control over the Federal Reserve at all. The reason it was called the Federal Reserve was that two previous attempts to create a central bank of the United States had already been forced to collapse by the will of the American people. So, it was suggested by Warburg that these men call it something else, the Federal Reserve System, instead of calling it what it actually is, which is a United States central bank. From its inception, there was an intent to conceal the truth that it is not a federal entity.

This was only the beginning of the plan of these men. They systematically devised a plan to always keep the American people behind the proverbial eight ball and never allow the average person to ascend into their ranks of wealth. They first wanted to initiate the concept of deficit spending into every household, in other words, buy now, pay later. In order to do so, they conceptualized a four-step policy to force all people into such a mentality and really set the pattern of financial destruction plaguing us even to this day.

The four main points that they came up with were: 1) being able to always crush the competition; 2) how to control interest rates, which leads into 3) how controlling the interest rates would enable them to be able to make as many loans as they wanted, regardless of how much money they had to actually back up all of those loans. The biggest one was 4) that they knew that this was essentially a Ponzi scheme and would inevitably crash, maybe many times, and that when that happened, they needed a safeguard so that they and their banks would not be held responsible or financially accountable and, most importantly, that the taxpayers, not the bank financiers, would be the ones having to actually pay back the remaining bill. This was not just the beginning of too big to fail; it also meant they would never see any type of come up pence or jail time resulting from any form of prosecution.

These were manipulative individuals who did not show much, if any, morality and were brilliant propagandists who have given birth to the unfortunate culture we have now in the world, where being morally bankrupt is somehow now something to overlook or apparently even strive to attain. This is where the fall of Western civilization was created, bringing us to the tipping point that we now currently live in, where money has become more important than morality, forsaking all integrity. Greed is not good. Greed precedes the fall.

J.P. Morgan was known for handing out shiny dimes to people on the street; of course, what is a shiny dime versus all the dirty money that was formulated from his policies that still endure to this day? Paul Warburg was the basis for Daddy Warbucks in Little Orphan Annie, used to propagandize a totally false reality versus the man who corrupted the American Dream for over the past 115 years, to today. Social media was not the beginning of creating a false reality of appearance for those who have so much, and, in fact, the ideas and basis of most creative image consultants today are based even now on these false realities that were created so long ago. The false image projected by so many who have power and influence now has replaced the soul for far too many, corrupting society.

One of the most influential banks that Paul Warburg used for the creation of the Federal Reserve, which once again is still in use in the United States of America to this day, was the Reichsbank, which gave Adolf Hitler the ability to rise to power in Germany. The Reichsbank was a central banking system, just like the Federal Reserve, that gave birth to massive hyperinflation, decreased the purchasing power of the currency, collapsed its economy, and crushed the German middle class. What most people are not aware of in history is that a director who ran the Reichsbank in Germany was Paul Warburg's brother, Max Warburg. A theory has been espoused often since the onset of World War I that it was Max Warburg, as the head of M.M. Warburg in Hamburg, Germany, who purportedly advised Kaiser Wilhelm prior to the war. It has been theorized by some that the brothers financed the war from different sides of the conflict. This may have always been the plan all along.

No wonder Nelson Aldrich never sent any notes to the United States of America from his trip abroad to learn how to fix the economy and banking system. The formulation of these policies was most likely the plan from its inception and was set in motion by the meeting at Jekyll Island in Georgia after a train trip from Hoboken, New Jersey, that carried all of the most influential men from New York City to the destiny that they created for all of us, which still impedes the ability of every single American's life today to flourish financially.

The reason that the entire world is still affected even today by these men and their creation, the Federal Reserve, is that the dollar of the United States of America is the world's reserve currency, and any inflation created by the Federal Reserve is felt around the entirety of Earth. Also, there is the undeniable reality that the United States of America's government spends much more every year than it brings in. This is still the exact concept of deficit spending created at Jekyll Island in Georgia. The government of the United States of America then makes up some of the difference by selling Treasury bonds. If and when the Federal Reserve increases the money supply, such as through cryptocurrency or printing money, then the dollars that bondholders are being paid back with are essentially worth less than their value at the time of purchase. This means that even the bond investors are being taken advantage of, unless, of course, they are complicit and doing so knowingly in advance.

Ned Lamont, the current governor of Connecticut, is the grandson of J.P. Morgan's right-hand man, who even became J.P. Morgan's spokesperson for the man himself when J.P. Morgan was retiring. Eventually, Thomas Lamont was the acting head of J.P. Morgan, the company, on Black Thursday in 1929, when the stock market crashed. That day's event is often considered the proximate cause of the Great Depression. There is a question as to whether Thomas Lamont orchestrated the financial collapse on purpose. Some feel that this is the most likely scenario. This is due to the fact that President Herbert Hoover had previously contacted Lamont about his concerns about the constant market manipulation by Wall Street insiders that was rampant and the financial risks it created for the average American working-class citizen invested in the stock market. Lamont responded flippantly, stating, "The future appears brilliant," to President Herbert Hoover. The market crashed the following Thursday, October 24, 1929, and the crash was exacerbated the following Tuesday, October 29, 1929. Billions of dollars of investment were wiped out in hours, triggered by mass panic.

Also of importance is the fact that it was later discovered that Thomas Lamont had kept a preferential stock list for certain clients of J.P. Morgan, which allowed those clients to liquefy their stocks during the crash at premium prices compared to actual stock market value. This list included prominent bankers, other people of influence, and politicians, including at least one person who would go on to become president of the United States of America.

Thomas Lamont was one of the company's most important and influential men abroad prior to this event as well. Lamont had become a partner at J.P. Morgan & Co. in 1911. He would become chairman of the board of J.P. Morgan, the company, after the man J.P. Morgan died. Lamont played a large role in making 1913 the year that serfdom was created for all United States citizens who were not rich, in a system of debt creation that still exists to this day. He was a member of the Jekyll Island Club on Jekyll Island in Georgia.

There were two main creations of policy that have influenced finance in the United States of America and the rest of the world ever since and both actions of government occurred in 1913. The year 1913 was the year of the creation of the Federal Reserve Bank in the United States and also the year the 16th Amendment was passed, that took the United States away from tariffs that provided income for the federal government and made it so that United States citizens would be taxed for the first time ever with a federal income tax. Many people then and now consider the taxation of Americans a system that has held back the people from being able to move forward or even to exist at a higher plane during the course of their lifetimes.

The 16th Amendment granted the federal government the power to levy taxes, and the Federal Reserve was established under a separate agreement. Those two acts of legislative action, created by people who wanted to maintain their own individual power and strengthen their ability to grow their financial strength regardless of how those acts impacted the vast majority of the population, have dominated the financial landscape of the United States of America and the world economy ever since. It was then that taxes replaced tariffs as the way the government paid to subsidize its own operational expenditures and to invest in future programs to provide infrastructure for the citizens of the country. The collection of large pools of money that often go unaccounted for has led to rumors of rampant waste, fraud, and abuse of the tax funds collected ever since. The American people have very little say in how this money is distributed. Often, programs are designed to help specific demographics of people instead of the entire collective citizenry as a whole unit of people.

This led the American government to create a new form of economic development and eventually was a major cause of the removal of the gold standard in the 1970s. There were a tremendous number of smart people who were against this action occurring and tried to reverse the course of the action afterwards. Once again, many people hold strong convictions that this additional act during the 1970s further separated the people who hold power and wealth from the rest of the people in the citizenry of the United States of America who do not hold such prestige in wealth or power. There is a belief that, while all were affected, this was done by a central group of authorities who were ensuring their ability to maintain control over the masses and prevent any possible action of financial institutions being overtaken by the people. Generations have lived in this format ever since. We still do today.

There is a plan to correct the financial state that currently exists, and it includes paying off all of the bondholders, which would allow the United States of America to get rid of the Federal Reserve. The plan gets rid of all debt, and then people are able to start again without the games for we the people, not we the rich. While theoretically possible, it is probably not realistic due to the volatility of worldwide foreign financial dependency on the U.S. dollar. The unintended consequences could be disastrous. If a situation arises that does allow for this idea to be possible, with the ability to diminish conceivable negative repercussions in advance, then maybe this can become an idea to be utilized. However, this concept may only occur after completely investigating the pros and cons of whether such a measure should be initiated to begin with and the long-term ramifications that could prove to be deleterious.

The reason all of this is relevant is that we are living in the day and age of monopolies. These conglomerate companies can control how wealth is distributed among the masses of people. There is no true capitalism anymore, as there is no, or at least very limited, competition in the marketplace. The domino effect of big box stores taking out Main Street businesses has quickly caused the financial landscape in the United States of America to devolve to the point that there is almost no possibility of living the American Dream anymore. Those big box stores were bought up, and then fewer, and then even fewer, businesses were able to survive the new landscape of power that existed. Within only a few decades, this has led to a limited number of corporations being able to influence the pattern of business development.

BlackRock, State Street, and Vanguard have taken over a major portion of finance within the United States. It is estimated that these three companies are among the top five shareholders of nearly 70% of the 2,000 largest publicly traded firms in the United States of America. The world's largest investment firm is BlackRock, which manages over $12.5 trillion in assets.xviii Even these companies are prone to having economic climate shifts, such as when a single client in Asia withdrew $52 billion. BlackRock has made significant investments in Europe, especially Great Britain, and purchased Global Infrastructure Partners and HPS.xix

The owners of Uber and Lyft are essentially the same companies. The owners of Uber Eats and DoorDash are essentially the same corporations and the same businesses that own Uber and Lyft. BlackRock and Vanguard also own a large majority of shares in Disney, as majority stakeholders, and almost all, if not all, of the holdings underneath Disney, such as McDonald's. This also brings to pass questions about Disney's upcoming plans for new development of propulsion motors and how its animatronics are utilized. Could these devices be weaponized under various conditions? BlackRock, State Street, and Vanguard own a large number of these devices and other devices that theoretically could be used for purposes such as thought implementation and the extraction of thoughts. BlackRock, State Street, and Vanguard financially back each other and appear to own most of each other too.

This has also led to these companies owning various media stations that have led to mass propaganda distribution rather than actual news reporting. While there is no governing body for registered classification for news stations, the pursuit of profits by these supposed news channels, hastened in the 1980s has resulted in a reality where there are no longer qualified news stations as most people would define them or expect them to uphold the news to a certain standard of measurable truth. These stations are now news entertainment channels. It does not appear that the Federal Communications Commission (FCC) often investigates false claims of information. The standards of conduct concerning truth and the news from Edward R. Murrow have been forgotten and no longer seem to apply. From newspapers to television to the internet, mass propaganda is infecting society, and it seems this propaganda is not permitting the truth to be told anywhere by anyone at any time consistently. When one group becomes dominant, it becomes difficult for others to survive. Sometimes, though, the little one can stand up to the dominant, bigger group and create a place for themselves; this may be that chance with this health care program.

Processed food leading to weight gain is a concern, as obesity has been on the rise for many years now. It turns out that companies like BlackRock, State Street, Vanguard, Unilever, Nestlé, and PepsiCo are heavily invested in and involved in both the ultra-processed food market and the health care sector. These are companies that are making money off of producing goods and services that tend to create obesity and other health conditions and then are also heavily interested in the health care industry for marketing purposes with various products and services.

A major additional concern is that the government of the United States of America continues to kick the can down the road financially, which keeps putting unbelievable pressure on future generations to be able to survive. The Congressional Budget Office indicates that a recently passed bill will create about five trillion dollars per year; however, the same bill will generate incredible debt as well, as there will now be a need for seven trillion dollars in spending per year. The average American family is considered to be $230,000 in debt; the new bill will have that rise to $425,000 per household within the next 10 years.[xx] [xxi] This increase in debt raises more questions about hyperinflation and continued devaluation of the dollar. It also raises the possibility that future generations will be handed a check by this current generation that will be impossible to cash. Major reforms that cut spending, increase income, and create positive deflation are necessary right now.

The day of the penny candy has long since expired. Hopefully, inflation is currently stabilized; however, the rate at which inflation has been steadied is still incredibly disconcerting. We must examine things from a worst-case scenario, not a best-case scenario that may never materialize. Fluctuations in the marketplace could lead to something that goes awry. If something does go wrong, it is possible that even a mid-level event could lead to global financial collapse. This concern is worsened due to the current political climate, which could lend itself to chaos domestically and worldwide, unfortunately.

The perversion of Walden Pond and the transcendentalist movement ideals of the authors, versus today's reality of what has happened to Walden Pond near Boston, Massachusetts, is an unfortunate example of expectations of a lived lifestyle versus the reality of long-term financial gain possibilities. The entire point of the transcendentalist authors and poetry movement was to rail against the necessities of technology and especially finance ruling our lives completely. The point was that happiness comes from living in nature and not succumbing to the world of capitalist concerns of economic importance. In reality, after the authors died, so did their lifestyle and point. Economics affect everyone all over Earth.

Inevitably, the bubble will burst, no matter what. Everything you know will cease to exist in the way that you are currently aware of how things work. The question is, do you want to have any chance of having any control over how things work if that burst bubble were to exist and become real very soon? Unfortunately, it appears that this financial volatility needed to be proven as part of functional math before the analysis of financial equations concerning these worrying issues. In other words, this all occurred before we decided to evaluate the reality of circumstances. How long will it take, and what will it take, before remedial action is enacted and applied? Will it take an irreversible economic disaster before you take action?

There need to be positives of reality in the economic forecast for that revitalization to occur. Doing so will also provide a solid foundation for future financial prospects as well, both in the United States of America and throughout the entire world. So, how do we fix it so that we can all have a chance at a fair share to eat at the dinner table in the future? Instituting this new health care plan and all of its phases may be our only conceivable method for now.

Additionally, in order to invigorate economic opportunities, a prime example would be North Carolina lithium production, which would then be utilized for the creation of commercial chips developed domestically. This would take away the United States of America's dependency on Nvidia and also drastically reduce the need to buy these chips from China. In addition, the United States of America would immediately become a viable competitor in the marketplace to produce the best computer processing chips in the world.

Being able to produce those chips domestically would also have positive repercussions that would permit new job growth and, eventually, entirely new industries that would permit the United States of America to become the world leader in various inventive industries that will transform and revolutionize the health industry and other businesses as well. An all-inclusive nanotechnological data transponder containing all pertinent information, from health to finance, will replace the need for wallets and identification cards and will even be internally regulated. These passports will change the landscape of all future business transactions, health requirements, and the need for identification purposes.

Those who do not know history are doomed to repeat it. The stock market being falsely propagated by the industrial complex dependent on war means peace cannot occur for them to turn a profit. If that market were to be taken away, the speculative marketplace might crash overnight. This would lead to a run on stock sales, which would depreciate the value of all stocks and lead to vulnerability in the security of the US dollar, which would then affect all global marketplaces and currencies worldwide, as the dollar is the currency that all other currencies are based on. That market fluctuation could cause further distrust in investments, leading to a global economy faltering even worse than it did during the Great Depression, with this time there being a possibility of no recovery occurring at all. Some who tried to displace the US dollar during Covid are now dependent on the USA fixing its economy to avoid major upheaval among the citizens of their own countries, an uproar that could result in the downfalls of governments and even countries ceasing to exist.

Even in the United States of America, what was the point of fighting and dying for freedom only to sell out major companies and our land to foreign investors? This has literally sold out the American Dream for most people alive today and those who will be tomorrow. The system in place currently of the Federal Reserve was meant to prevent the ability of the common person from having the ability to obtain the wealth and power of these patriarchal families that have controlled the US and world economy ever since. There is no freedom in that concept. The problems of foreign lands from which our immigrants escaped have followed them here to the US, not because of them but because of the infrastructure of the USA being sold out to foreign investors, many of which do not pay taxes in any way, shape, or form to the US government now. The real estate market has been left especially vulnerable due to this reality, as many commercial and home real estate properties are being purchased by major conglomerate companies, not individual middle class families that are from the United States of America. Some of these countries may be the same ones responsible for Covid and purposeful economic and sociological warfare perpetrated within the United States of America before, during, and since the inception of the Covid epidemic.

It is possible Covid was an attempt by the players of the world as part of an arranged alliance to eradicate this current financial system; however, since it was done by force and was, by all accounts, a deadly, negative, passive aggressive force, the attempted financial coo failed completely because the motive was not peace; it was greed. This action led to the downfall of many of those other nations' economies, fittingly. Corruption due to narcissism and greed around the world from other countries, including some of the United States' most aggressive adversaries throughout the past century, including Germany, China, and other Central European countries that also have been thought to be our allies, may have been complicit.

Now, all the world needs the economy of the United States to recover, even flourish, so that other economies throughout the world may have an opportunity to recover and improve themselves. Ironically, even the countries and people involved in the issue of the economic coo now need the United States to rebound financially so that those other countries may revitalize their economic possibilities in the future as well. This even includes the countries that are thought of as being adversarial to the interests of the United States of America.

This has left us with quite a dilemma to fix within the United States of America, and it affects every living person in the entire world as well. Since many of the financiers that were responsible for creating the Federal Reserve were and still are mostly families foreign to the USA, the question must be asked: Was this the plan all along? Was the freedom earned by the United States of America during the Revolutionary War sold out after the United States of America fought to end slavery internally and worldwide? Was this when it was decided that, regardless of race, ethnicity, or religion, the middle class of the United States of America would be a working class of a constant slave state for all people? This leads us to the most important questions of all: What are we going to do to correct this issue now? Also, the follow up question: What will we do to ensure that this is never possible to occur again so that financial stability permits health to be of paramount importance for every single person who is alive today and who will ever be? Today is the time to take action and create a better, healthier existence for all of us. Now is the time. Some people must ask themselves whether they will continue to stand for irrelevant matters or stand for what is truly important. Are you ready to take action now? The new word for love is yes, and compassionate action of positivity is the method to take. Say yes to yourself and all of existence now. Say yes and mean that love is important to you, society, the entire world, and the whole of existence throughout the universe for all eternity.

Do not be dissuaded by false rhetoric that is designed purposefully to weaponize you against yourself and others.

The delusions of importance applied are only there to maintain power for those who have always had it and to ensure that you fight against yourself so you will never have that type of wealth, power, prestige, and, most important, influence in the future. Would you prefer to shape the future or be ruined today by those who stole the promise from it yesterday? This is meant to incite passion for directed purpose, not war. Peace must be our objective and best weapon to achieve a global concept of health for all.

When we work our way forward and are able to improve the economic situation of the world, we all will enjoy life more and spend less. The reality is, when we do, there is a distinct possibility to examine new thought patterns of how to exist. When this is done, there are definitely green pastures ahead of us on the horizon, and the harvest from the fields we seed will become an overwhelmingly bountiful yield and permit crops of the future to have a much more stable foundational point of having the nutrients necessary to live well and prosper for generations to come. The light is on and will be shining brightly, illuminating so that we may see as far as possible once we endeavor to fix the realities of concern that some currently deny exist.

Beware of faulty foundations, as they can lead to misleading results that may require a great deal of time passing before the consequences are felt. When they are felt, they most likely lead to the feeling of wishing one had done things in a professional manner with the appropriate applications necessary to begin with. What good is a beautiful home if it is built on a faulty foundation? The implementation of a new health care policy aids in generating immediate financial stabilization. Both are necessities for providing the requisite preliminary, fundamental, foundational promise that creates real opportunities that will promote long-term stability and health as a portion of all parts of human existence.

There are many other concerns that we will inevitably be faced with very shortly. We will also have to deal with those concerns together, does not work to help us advance. Sorry to Thespis de Milito; however, this is not something that we can act our way out of. This requires real, true action right now without hesitation. In addition, we may only have a few opportunities, possibly only this one, so let us endeavor to make sure that this takes place as soon as possible and with as much unity as possible during the initial implementation and always thereafter as well, regardless of how difficult it is, for it will always be worth it for everyone. Let us not wait for the collective pond to cause deadly disease before starting a clean water endeavor or procrastinate until after the pollution in our atmosphere makes it impossible to have a breath of fresh air. Let us also make sure the allocated funds for such a promising, positive project are directly utilized and used correctly without delay.

People acting as ostriches, sticking their heads into the dirt, and others not being meek but acting weak like sheep does not work. We need to invigorate a healthy mindset of mind, body, and soul, and this shall ignite the biggest financial and spiritual comeback in history. The healthy team usually wins in the playoffs. The Captain America, Captain Comeback, Roger Staubach Hail Mary is needed right now, and it shall be completed if we are willing to take the necessary steps as soon as possible. Instead of looking with doom and gloom at tomorrow, we may find a way to end our careers with home runs in our last at bats like Ted Williams and provide optimism to all who follow so that they may do the same.

The American Dream is not dead; it just needs to be resuscitated. The United States is still a beautiful country where you can start with nothing and achieve everything. The dreams of our youth may not materialize the way we would hope; however, doors will open and paths can be followed that allow each of us to discover incredible success in life. America is still the land of opportunity. While happiness may never be guaranteed, the pursuit of that happiness still is a vibrant part of the fabric of America. Good luck occasionally occurs and generally does when one is prepared for an opportunity. We must venture forth and create good luck by maximizing our opportunities in every facet of existence throughout the entire Universe for the rest of time. We must band together and find our path that makes dreams reality for the majority of the population. Destruction is easy; constructive behavior is hard, takes time, and is full of obstacles, and yet, so rewarding when achieved that it can be overwhelming with the emotion of earned accomplishment that it fills our hearts with a sense of joy and inspiration that makes the entire endeavor worth it in every possible way.

In order to revive the economy, we must be willing to do what is necessary in order to position ourselves so that tomorrow morning, our financial forecast will shine brightly. Also, the ideas implemented must be based on opportunities that are real for solid financial growth without increasing deficits and causing more inflation. The concepts provided currently do not address this. The reality is this plan will help. Deflation resulting in a higher efficiency of the value of the dollar and the purchasing power of the dollar, and of all other currencies, is possible now if the proper methodology is implemented and adhered to.

Value for the dollar, the purchase power of the dollar, can be revitalized, and the momentum gained will provide encouraging results that provide the evolutionary basis for constructive ideas tomorrow as well. Positive deflation due to job growth in entirely new industries that are far more lucrative than today's current marketplace will actually permit the purchasing power of the dollar to buy much more than it has in years. We will make the pennies count again; do not throw them out. While the wishes we make may still be worth more in the interim, the inevitable nature is that they may not in the end. It is a good bet that we will gain positive momentum, and the returns on investment will be expedited exponentially with every little positive step we take and make for the foreseeable future.

Creative scientific animation models for all services will immediately become available that will provide many good years to come in a variety of industries by forecasting the maximum possible efficiency capable of being achieved at that moment and demonstrating appropriately what we can chase and achieve as realistic, obtainable dividends as we will be the builders of tomorrow today. These models will provide vivid imagery leading to detailed creations for all industries, education, and all available applications. These will be on budget forecast models individualized for each and every industry. All businesses will have an opportunity to thrive again, not just struggle to survive.

We will create a cohesive balance sheet of financial opportunities that demonstrate a wide range of diversity and integration of international diplomacy that will potentially provide possible opportunities for peaceful development of diplomatic measures that help to encourage the reduction of both domestic and international conflicts while immediately helping aid all peaceful actions that will substantiate a long-term positive yield of growth of all sorts, including financial, on an exponential level for good in a worldwide and eventually intergalactic market place that encourages financial viability and opportunity for all people alive on this planet now and on any planet inhabited in the future as well.

CHAPTER 12

SAFETY & SECURITY

Implementation of security programs necessary to protect medical information going forward will need to be far better than what is currently available. Even modern Pentagon level technology is not sufficient. We must secure safety in our medical settings, especially in concern to medical records.

Verification for personal identification security should always be done in real time. All security access should have at least a double check methodology applied to be completed within a certain window of time. The security for the keeping of all health records for all human beings on Earth using artificial intelligence, as well as all access to any data, needs to be protected with the implementation of engineering standards that are state of the art. It is imperative that the system be impenetrable.

Security for the system that grants access to and protects all health care records, all medical information, and all pertinent billing data for insurance, hospitals, and doctors should be Pentagon level or better at inception to promote safeguarding and prevent weaponization of artificial intelligence and the health care system. This is important because a simple peanut allergy could prove to be deadly if someone were to hack in and replace the appropriate data with false information. All people need to know they are safe from such a predatory attack; this is especially true if the patient is a current world leader.

The Defense Advanced Research Projects Agency is responsible for security techniques that have been employed in various manners worldwide throughout the past seventy years. DARPA may be able to provide solutions to the security problem that need to be implemented immediately to ensure proper security for all devices and accumulated data. DARPA is considered to be on the cutting edge of technology and defense capabilities currently. They may have identified strengths and weaknesses of security protocols that may facilitate protection of all pertinent data networks necessary to protect the long-term viability of this project. In addition, they may be able to provide short-term protection while the system is being created for long-term sustainable usage and initiatives that will follow.

We need pragmatic cloud services that enable and protect while providing the platform necessary for data accrual and protection of all information accumulated. The leading global chip fabrication companies will be necessary for the creation and distribution of all necessary chips and software to be able to initiate implementation improvements immediately in response to all possible problems and consequences we currently need to address. In addition, it would be helpful to immediately start large scale chip creation domestically within the United States of America.

Safeguarding information is an important factor in all forms of all aspects of this entire process. The only things that are more important to safeguard are our homes, communities, and especially our families. Essentially, the data centers of importance will be an impenetrable safe for medical information management for a database that holds all of the world's information on all people.

The database will be a key container for all artificial intelligence security of all health insurance records and information. Safeguard record centers already exist. The capabilities they have will be useful, including role-based access controls concerning information. The technology they are currently employing, though, is about to become totally obsolete instantaneously when artificial intelligence integrates new ideas and concepts never before imagined, such as biomass security.

Guarding record keeping information at various record maintenance storage facilities will be required. Guarding such information will be of economic importance and require extensive, experienced electronic management teams, including elite specialists in various industries. Fiberoptic laser surveillance enhanced with optical ability for immediate facial recognition constantly applied to all who are permitted to enter secure facilities will be mandatory at all such places. Biomass requirements will also be mandatory at all facilities of storage.

It is even possible that nanotechnology could play a role as well, especially if it could be integrated into a rotational looping system of codes over a multisystem layered network. To do so will require multiple different artificial intelligence operating systems integrated into one cohesive unit that regulates biomass, numbers, and proper chronology with sequencing that is updated every five to ten minutes so as to eliminate all possibility of the system being compromised and to eliminate any and all possibility of any threats at all. If that time can be enhanced for proper sequencing to be changed even faster, while still maintaining some semblance of human ability to recover and control the system if catastrophe strikes, then that ideal number of timings per hour of chronological sequencing should be adhered to moving forward. The symbiotic element has to be necessitated for human involvement while permitting artificial intelligence to thrive and defend in all new ways. Quantum mechanics should also be employed and will be helpful. This system can then be utilized for security in all aspects of life with all matters of import.

In other words, security would be about timing in addition to number coding, like an alarm system or bank ATM code, and additionally could require biomass procedures, including but not limited to, DNA and RNA in addition to actual body mass being calculated periodically and updated as necessary to even access data or for utilization of home security and for accessing all monetary funds. This should eliminate most crimes of theft and impersonation. A new cypher language for coding will also be necessary and used in conjunction with artificial intelligence on multiple platforms to disguise all information. All previous forms of encryption may be utilized in a meaningful manner of cohesive cooperation; however, they will most likely be extinct as individual pathways in the future.

There are some main forms of artificial intelligence to be utilized in a rotational real time access method where windows of security time apply. Possible inclusions of various forms of existing artificial intelligence would be Cassandra, Pi AI, Claude, Gemini and Gotham. A second layer should also be embedded so crime is nearly impossible. From the Alpha to the Omega, a new language of source engineering may be necessary for truly providing the security necessary to protect the information of all members of the medical database.

In concern to an artificial intelligence looping security system, if necessary, a third layer of security can be added. If there is ever a security breach somehow constructed in the future to penetrate those layers, infinite layers may be added by artificial intelligence; however, symbiotic requirements with human beings should always be maintained.

Only certain systems can handle such information and the volume of information. Security teams at Access or Google may already have identified potential security enhancements. Palantir's two main operating systems are Gotham and Foundry. Gotham is an artificial intelligence platform that helps governments collect data and is helpful in planning various missions, including usage of satellites and utilization of drones used for surveillance, plus data accumulation and analysis.

Gotham may be required to help navigate the system correctly. Foundry may provide additional opportunities for data collection, analysis, assessment, and quality improvement. Cassandra is another open-source artificial intelligence that may be able to provide useful information on how to maintain and protect the integrity of stored information as well as encrypted communications. With the advent of integrated artificial intelligence and its constant improvements, there is a possibility that the assimilation of all other artificial intelligence programs, such as Pi AI, Claude, Gemini, and other operating systems, will allow them all to work together in a system that performs optimally, providing prime efficiency.

Quantum may be a requirement to think about as a potential security issue moving forward in concern to all developments for safety and security in the future. Essentially, regardless of what instrumentation is created using artificial intelligence for safety and security now, it is theoretically possible that in the future, quantum could act like a battering ram and discover a way to overcome all current and newly developed safeguards. Using quantum theories may be, and probably is, necessary in reality to safeguard all medical information immediately. Integrating quantum theories, including the application of quantum mechanics, may become a necessity now for all security measures moving forward forever. Quantum mechanics is already being utilized in various fields of technology, including medicine, lasers, global positioning satellites, smartphones, computers, and much more.

There are tremendous concerns about security in the current financial marketplace. Both impersonation that leads to people taking out loans against homes they do not own and financial theft of epic proportions that is easier than ever are very real concerns that jeopardize financial wellbeing. Computer programmers from various countries have been a cheap form of labor compared with those in the United States for many years now. While call centers are what most people think of first, there are many computer engineering and programming jobs that have been done abroad for many years now. The coding and sequencing by some of these engineers in other countries have been dubious at best.

There are times in some programmers' coding when back doors are created that permit the theft of information and direct theft from bank accounts. Many times, these are not even capable of being noticed, and at times now, they are created by the same people claiming to be the ones providing security on computers, the internet, and even for major financial corporations. Often, the information found through these backdoor access points is used to be able to put those programmers in positions of leverage that are far more lucrative than directly stealing money from an account. Having information on an individual that the person does not want to become known can influence their decision making and integrity.

Hacking into video surveillance at theme parks has never been easier for certain people. Data collection has led to a new age of criminals. This theft occurs from offices of local insurance brokers, medical professionals, lawyers, and most common neighborhood businesses. Sometimes, even major institutions and companies have been breached for their information. The people committing these acts go from local hackers all the way to nefarious gangs and organized crime. Many times, local officers and governmental law enforcement have been compromised due to information that has been collected on them, which puts them in situations where their value systems are conceded, sometimes willingly, sometimes to protect those they care about most.

Awful staff at places with public services has become a major issue, and this cannot happen when those services are being provided to protect and serve the public at large. This means that there has been an infiltration of negativity into our police and fire forces on an individual level that has also had a deleterious effect on our armed services as well, including special programs of the local and federal government responsible for major investigations. It is time to clean up this issue right now. The extensive criminality that exists in the majority of society has taken hold everywhere. While some years have passed now, the names Aldrich Ames and Robert Hanssen demonstrate how even the most trusted may not be worthy of being trusted at all. The odds are now that most corruption would be for corporations, wealthy individuals, and some organizations over countries. It is time to realize the concept of addition by subtraction; trash removal cleans up the environment.

There are serious ethical concerns in the fields of security and safety that are very real now. Rampant criminality has become too much of a part of everyday lives for all children now. Since Covid began, the level of safety and security throughout the entire USA has diminished. The effect of the National Guard being sent into various regions has shown how dramatically the idea of true law enforcement can cause crime rates, especially violent crime rates, to drop. It does make one wonder why this method has been so effective in lowering violent crime rates where employed. The police in those areas may have been outmatched. Were they?

There appears to be such fecund corruption in the police across the entire nation now that it is hard to find officers that live up to the motto of protecting and serving the citizenry. Defunding the police has resulted in a horrendous state where it seems mostly only the officers that are profiting illegally have remained. In fact, there has been an incredibly high level of retirements occurring within most levels of most police departments in recent years. This has apparently left the cupboard barren of decent individuals performing the noble profession of being a police officer honorably. It has become difficult in many instances to see where the criminal ends and the member of law enforcement begins, as in too many cases around the country, they have become the same entity. Unfortunately, this has led to a situation where the good guy and the bad guy are the exact same person; the cop has too often willingly become the crook. This has also made it difficult for the honorable officers to stay safe.

There are still wonderful people undertaking a call of duty to protect and serve the public. Unfortunately, the job has become much more dangerous for these good people because of the danger involved inherently in this line of work being exacerbated by crooked brothers and sisters. Of course, officers are individuals like anyone else in any other profession; however, due to the power construct in which weaponry is legally used by police, immediate corrective action is necessitated for all levels of law enforcement throughout the entire country of the USA. Lethal means are only justifiable for a member of law enforcement when no other means are available. Shooting out a tire on a car or wounding someone in the leg allows for justice to still be carried out in a court system, although the courts need to be cleaned too. The levels of power flexing their administrative muscle for selfish purposes are now normal. It starts with corruption within our government organizations. What are children left to think if the very people that they regard as heroes are the villains?

When artificial intelligence robots start working with the police in a symbiotic relationship, it will reflect a tried-and-true principle that has been in place for years. Trained police dogs are officially officers pursuant to laws in most states, and they put themselves in harm's way by often running point when trying to track a suspect and putting their lives on the line. They are usually the ones called in to help with certain investigations, as they frequently augment the abilities of the human officers with abilities that humans do not have, like a super sense of smell. Often, in dangerous situations, a police dog is the one whose life is risked first. The idea of officers working together in a symbiotic relationship is nothing new and has been proven effective time and time again. Robotic officers will do the same, as they will be augmenting the human forces with special abilities and reducing risk for human officers and firefighters by assuming actions responsibly as necessary in dangerous situations.

It is highly unlikely that human beings will be used as much in the future as police, firefighters or soldiers. There will always be a need for the best of the best with the most integrity and abilities to be part of a symbiotic relationship of security to protect and serve all communities all over the world and even as we traverse throughout the Universe. For the most part, though, robotic technology will replace many of the more dangerous undertakings currently performed by humans. All integrated artificial intelligence robotics, from police officers to air support, will be able to function with precision, synchronized timing, and capabilities that are far beyond what human beings are presently capable of performing. Firefighting, search and rescue, and saving people from disasters will be able to be done on an entirely different level. Imagine a child stuck on the third floor of a burning building that is difficult, if not impossible, for humans to enter due to the scope of the fire, and a robot that simply jumps up into the fire and puts the child inside its skeleton, with a heat-resistant shield providing protection with padding. Then the robot, while providing immediate burn therapy remedies, if necessary, jumps back to the ground and releases the child from within into the grateful arms of the child's mom and dad.

Fewer human troops will be utilized in the military in the near future as the robotics industry continues to improve. The evolution in artificial intelligence has already led to various possibilities for robot soldiers with safety mechanism functionality. This has been seen in soldier training videos from many countries which have been available online to anyone at any time for many years now. There will always be a need and a place for the bravest, smartest, and the most courageous among us as human beings with a duty to protect all life forms with a sense of integrity and a heart that encourages peace, love, and prosperity for all life.

There may be brand new security measures to even start your car, withdraw money from the bank, or be able to access your house as well. This could involve the use of a nanotechnology encrypted passport biomedically injected as a necessary component for all infrastructure information for everyone. While the terms are synonymous, we can use the term passport as a necessary term instead of the term transponder. People may access passport identification software, so security encryption and biometric security identification will have to be utilized simultaneously as safety measures for all individuals all over the world.

The transponders will enhance all current payment methods, from cash to PayPal, Venmo, and all the systems currently used. Using nanotechnology, the same technology used for mapping the synaptic firing within the human brain as well as monitoring and regulating other medical functions of the human body, may lead to massive reductions in crime and even possibly the eradication of theft.

Bio weight masses will be implemented and used for protection regarding possible abuse by criminals. These biomass scales must have the right input of reality, not theory. An easy-to-understand example currently would be using a scale for a precooked weight rather than the actual cooked weight. Such information can throw off the entire application of the mechanism. This would need to be constantly updated to each human's current exact biomass reality. Doing so will provide additional theft protection. These items discussed are only the beginning of major, inevitable, necessary changes to security and safety mechanisms to protect life in all its forms. The future starts right now.

CHAPTER 13

PRESSURE CALIBRATION STUDIES

Pressure calibration should be a study on multiple levels. A level of homeostasis is important for proper balance in a variety of different areas of life. Proper homeostasis provides improved performance, extended quality of life, and a reduction in problems, and, when properly adjusted and configured correctly, helps us to excel. Most of the population assumes that it exists at a level of homeostasis; however, this is rarely the case. Proper pressure can be the difference between being balanced appropriately and peacefully versus exploding unexpectedly and in a disastrous fashion.

There need to be studies into the effects of pressure on the human body, on the environment, on the planet, in the universe, on one another, on the pressure we put on ourselves, and on other areas of life too. Pressure applies stress, and stress can lead to multiple negative consequences, including ramifications for our health. An example of this concept is that cortisol release is a direct contributor to stress within a human being. Reducing the amount of cortisol released is positive, and, as such, the ability to overcome pressures can lead to literal improvement in an individual's health.

For most human beings, pressure is a part of our daily lives and can be measured in many ways. Cars are a really good example of pressure. Pounds per square inch (PSI) is used for measuring static pressure. For instance, with automobiles, an internal combustion engine requires 10 pounds per square inch of oil pressure for every 1,000 revolutions per minute (RPM). RPM measures how many times the engine's crankshaft makes one full rotation every minute and how many times each piston goes up and down in its cylinder. When cold, most car tires should have a PSI in the 30s. It is generally recommended that tires for a sedan or small sports utility vehicle (SUV) have a low of 30 to a maximum of 36 PSI.

When it comes to maintaining pressure with various substances, there is usually an ideal rate of flow that is not so high that something could literally blow up and not so low that the system clogs and could cause the entire system to shut down temporarily or, even worse, permanently. Typically, pressure is measured to maintain safety, usually in fifteen second intervals, to reach one minute of information gathering when multiplied by four. There is generally a hypothesis of an ideal rate of efficiency based on the whole system's base requirements for each individual application, especially if there is a concern of contamination. Fluids are measured by determining volume over time. The measurement of pressure is often calculated in gallons per minute (GPM) in the United States or liters per minute (LPM) in other countries. For example, a maximum of 2.5 gallons per minute (GPM) every 15 seconds, or a maximum of 10 gallons per minute (38 LPM) of measured flow, marks the ideal for gas flow pressure homeostasis at certain gas stations.

While tank pumps generally require constant pressure systems, exceptional calibration in multitudes of different fields will require imagery resonance diagnostic capabilities. This will be important for pressure calibration studies of all sorts in various industries and for exceedingly different purposes. In life, pressure studies of our internal resonance are not just physical studies, they are, at times, mental and even spiritual studies as well. Often, these factors can be the causes of stress that affect our health even more than the physical internal resonance factors. All facets being healthy is optimal.

Measuring pressure calibration with a different form of gas, gastrointestinal gas, could show pressures that are causing damage internally in the body. Farting can be a very healthy activity. As long as your gastrointestinal system is gurgling and working, it is generally a good sign. Relieving intestinal pain caused by gas is usually more helpful when it occurs by passing through as a fart rather than as a burp. With stomach issues, burping can be beneficial as well, though. Holding in gas that wants to be released is not healthy.

In an abbreviated version of a study of gastroenterology, it is possible to see how even common gas within the body can cause catastrophic problems within the human body and can exacerbate other problems regarding other ailments. Bloating, distension, pain, cramping, and flatulence are all forms of discomfort that occur when there is an abnormality in the regular level of homeostasis within our own internal pressure calibration. That pressure is slightly different for each of us, as is our susceptibility to irregularities from hereditary background and proclivities for having such issues from past and present choices. Even body posture, positioning, and movement while a person is sleeping play a role in the amount and release of internal gas products. Each person's needs are different.

The alimentary tract is also known as the digestive tract or gastrointestinal tract, as the terms are all synonyms of one another. No matter which term a person or medical professional prefers, this tract includes the mouth, esophagus, stomach, small intestine, large intestine, rectum and anus. This tract is how the human body has the abilities necessary for the process of taking in food, digesting, absorbing nutrients, and eliminating waste products. Peristalsis is the term for digestion when it comes to normal functional processing in a normal digestive system. Reverse peristalsis occurs when a person throws up.

The medical term in Latin for gas in the human body is borborygmus, known as a rumbling noise, caused by the propulsion of gas through the intestines.xxii Iens rectum means going in the right direction, while distal means further away from the center. When a person has gas bubbles going in the right direction, further away from their stomach, continuing through their alimentary tract and going through the sphincter, this is known as a fart. So, the word fart in Latin could be phrased as borborygmus iens rectum per distalem sphincterem transiens. It is a lot easier to say fart, although it is not always easy for the digestive system to function properly and permit the passing of gas.

A commonplace practice for a physician is to examine whether a patient's gastrointestinal tract is functioning properly by listening to the resonance of the tympany by tapping on the abdominal region of the body to determine how much gas is truly involved and possibly trapped inside the patient's digestive walls. A similar methodology on the abdominal walls also may indicate whether a hiatal hernia is present. Compressing the patient's abdominal area may be helpful in determining an acute appendicitis issue, especially if there is no rebound effect in the patient. Pain and discomfort may accompany all of these maladies.

The upper esophageal sphincter connects the pharynx (throat) and the esophagus (feeding tube), which creates the swallowing reflex, and it is important that this process is not impeded. If the process is affected, it may cause people to choke and could cause them to choke to death unless the Heimlich maneuver is employed and successful.

The sphincter pylori is the sphincter that connects the stomach to the intestines through the duodenum, and its impairment can cause acid reflux. It works in conjunction with the sphincter of Oddi. The sphincter of Oddi also connects to the duodenum at the beginning of the small intestine and is where the appropriate levels of bile and pancreatic enzymes are introduced into the digestive process to help with the separation between nutrient absorption and the removal of waste products. The ileocecal sphincter is involved in the involuntary functioning and regulation of transporting waste products in the internal process of digestion from the small intestine to the large intestine.

The anal sphincters control defecation and are comprised of both involuntary and voluntary sphincter functions. The musculus sphincter ani internus and the musculus sphincter ani externus control the impulse and release of waste products at the end of the internal digestive process. One is involuntary in function; the other is voluntary, and the combination of the two regulates normal function and can lead to other issues such as incontinence.

Acid reflux occurs when acid from the stomach can go back into the esophagus and even back into the mouth at varying levels of severity. This is a frequent, normal diagnosis. When the lower esophageal sphincter is affected by normal wear and tear or even by a predisposition due to hereditary concerns, this can cause acid reflux in certain people. As the sphincter becomes worn from normal wear and tear, normally from the aging process, this has different effects on each person's inherent capabilities, on how effective their initial stomach digestion process is, and on how problematic the concern may be in the future. This reduces the likelihood of normal functioning over time. The loss or impediment of function leads to what has become a common diagnosis of acid reflux in many people. Over time, the situation can worsen or even become a more serious concern and, in certain cases, can lead to multiple problems.

GERD, or gastroesophageal reflux disease, can also lead to problems such as dysfunction, dysphagia, and constant upper body chest pain. It can be terminated by proper diet consumption. Hiatal hernias can be caused by an increase in pressure within the body cavity and may result in additional pressure being forced upon the individuals' other internal organs within the body cavity. When the stomach pushes through the diaphragm, it is usually a sign of irritation and irregularity.

Respiratory function is a necessity for survival. Alveolar pressure is more commonly known as intrapulmonary pressure. This is the pressure in the lungs that regulates breathing. The pressure of how a person's lungs work is directly related to atmospheric pressure. When a person is inhaling and breathing in oxygen, the pressure is referred to as negative, as the pressure in the lungs is lower than the atmospheric pressure present at that moment. Exhaling leads to what is referred to as positive pressure, as the pressure in the lungs is greater than the atmospheric pressure present in those moments. Inhaling is also known as inspiration, while exhaling is commonly referred to as expiration.

The intrapleural pressure is the pressure in the thoracic cavity that normally functions in the negative to maintain a lower pressure to keep the lungs expanded. The ability to inflate like a balloon is important for proper lung function, and this is known as elasticity. The difference between the alveolar pressure and the intrapleural pressure is denoted as the transpulmonary pressure, or the inflating force on the lung, and demonstrates how much the lung can function like a balloon. When there is high tension placed upon the alveoli (air sacs) due to a surface deficiency of the lung, this can cause the lung to collapse. If this is due to the lung having a lack of an adequate coating, or because the alveoli fill with fluid, this is known as atelectasis. Another term for a collapsed lung is a pneumothorax. A pneumothorax commonly occurs when air leaks into the space between the lung and the thoracic chest wall, causing a change in the stabilized pressure of the lung. The most common causes of this pressure change can come from both hereditary concerns and from immediate impacts upon the body. The causes can range from anything such as underlying lung disease, asthma, cystic fibrosis, pneumonia, and smoking to chest injuries, high altitude, and even deep-sea diving. All of them result in the same issue of a pneumothorax, a collapsed lung, due to a major shift in pressure within the void of the body. Constant analysis of the individual using nanotechnology could lead to seeing precursors that would help to diminish or even prevent the onset of such a medical emergency.

Cysts can cause abnormalities that affect the normal internal regulatory function of other internal systems such as the digestive process. The pressure calibration being affected by one issue can cause significant problems with the function of other necessary normal tasks of the human body. The internal regulatory process of one operating system in the body sometimes has a normal level of homeostatic function that is different from other internal functions of the human body. When one is altered, it may affect and alter other internal pressure systems within the body cavity.

For example, multiple sebaceous cysts in the groin area of a male can lead to several complications that could lead to further health consequences. These cysts are not always painful; however, they can lead to painful moments. The cysts themselves grow over time to contain voluminous amounts of blood and pus that can weigh multiple pounds. When the cysts explode, it is often a disgusting mess that takes hours and sometimes days to completely drain and can require several cleanings to completely disinfect the affected area.

When the cysts explode, they demonstrate how many other bodily functions have been and are being affected by the cysts. When the cysts grow, they result in increased pressure on other internal bodily organs. Upon exploding, they will drain. Initially, there can be blood that has become viscous as it has started to congeal into dark red coagulated blood, which shows how unhealthy these cysts are alone. Unfortunately, that is only the beginning, though. After the blood starts to drain, large amounts of fluid of a yellow nature also start to mix with the blood, and this can go on for hours before it becomes serosanguineous in nature. Then the other organs internally start to function differently as well.

Initially, urine flow immediately occurs, as the urine has been prevented from flowing normally due to the excess internal pressure. Next, the gastrointestinal system shows that it was affected by permitting gas to finally be released from the body cavity, and this happens more and more frequently as the other organs start to return to their normal placement within the body cavity. During the entire process, an increase in body temperature, even resulting in heavy sweating, may occur, especially during the initial phase when the cysts are exploding. This then permits a large amount of defecation to ensue, which had previously been halted because of the internal pressure and organs shifting positions. This process may go on for days, even weeks, before finally subsiding. Even worse, the process then repeats itself every few months, or sometimes even more regularly for certain people. The worst part is that modern insurance considers the surgery necessary to remove these cysts an elective procedure. It sometimes costs thousands of dollars to remove the cysts, so most people live in suffering and agony while the problem persists painfully until the cysts are removed. Fatigue, weakness, and occasional bouts of dizziness also sometimes accompany the draining cysts. Additionally, the cysts themselves may also impact the ability of a male to sustain an erection, too.

The internal pressure of feeling internal organs returning to their original positioning is also quite painful. It may be somewhat reminiscent of what women encounter during a menstrual cycle with their period in that the pressure increases to a point where it not only affects internal pressure but also places a large degree of pressure on the abdominal wall and can result in muscle pain. In the case of the cysts, even muscle tears may occur within the abdominal muscles. Heating pads have been quite helpful to women for years during this time, and now they are helpful to men, too.

For those questioning whether pressure can cause the compounding of various functions internally, understanding how a muscle tear can lead to nerve function damage is one possible explanation. There are several more interesting internal and external functions in different disciplines. The application of the concept may lead to an entirely different understanding of our own human experience now and how human evolution happened and is occurring.

These are just examples of pressure function and regulation within the human body. The truth is that pressure is always all around us as well. Whether it be atmospheric pressure or gravity, there is constant pressure at play on all life forms, including the planet itself. There need to be studies created and conducted to discover what affects the constant levels of pressure exerted upon all life forms and what effects they have upon each individual moving forward. It will be beneficial to investigate what complications may be induced by this constant force of nature and existence. It is possible that many different ailments and cures may be discovered by simply studying these overlooked yet already recognized phenomena.

Inquiries into how external and internal pressure can affect health may be helpful in determining how to regulate pressures so that health may be optimized for all people. In addition, it is very probable that these investigations will lead to finding and defeating mysteries that have been part of the medical landscape for years and that still plague us because answers are not readily available or understood. These studies may develop into entirely new examinations that provide those answers for certain diagnoses that still have few medical therapies or, in some cases, for which no remedies currently exist.

For instance, how does pressure calibration play a role in temperature regulation? Do pressure calibration issues play a role in the formation of different forms of cancer? Are there certain factors of internal pressure on organs that promote renal failure or maybe even cause lupus? Are there answers to the onset of multiple sclerosis or Lou Gehrig's disease (amyotrophic lateral sclerosis)? Do internal and external pressures affect cognitive functions, including all forms of dementia, including early onset dementia? Is Alzheimer's something that could be prevented? There are so many more possibilities, including this: If an ability is fine tuned to help with some forms of cognitive function disabilities, will those same findings be able to be used to enhance all cognitive abilities? Will it help for communication purposes with ourselves, with each other, and even with other learners from other planets if we were to encounter them in the future? Will these studies enable us to learn how to communicate in new ways? Simply put, if we are able to use these findings to defeat certain illnesses, diseases, and disabilities in life, we will then be able to utilize those findings to enhance the quality of each and every life moving forward for the rest of time.

The study of pressure calibration in a variety of fields will be so useful to so many people in so many different ways that it has to be discovered by exploring all concepts of application. This could revolutionize the field of health care by changing the environment and field of medicine, medical studies, and all forms of medicinal applications forever. It may have unlimited applications. It is important to continue these studies in all forms and realms of life.

CHAPTER 14

ENERGY FLOW

It is important for each of us to see life from a genuine environment of energy flow perspective based on veritas, not a false ideal, but a reality-based notion of creating continuity. The foundation of building continuity and creating consistency is effectively communicated information. This is important for a multitude of reasons, including maintaining coherence in communication and cohesion among fellow employees, government officials, and united citizens of every country, and unifying all countries in one single cause for all of us.

Doing the hard work in life is never easy. However, it is necessary, as most people frequently find that overcoming the difficulties of life creates inner strength, confidence and resilience. For those who have overcome adversity, these experiences become new foundations of life and permit each person to go through the ups and downs of their existence with each other and themselves with the greatest amount of information possible to be successful. In this case, winning against the adversities and difficulties of life may lead to every one of us enjoying living in the fast lane of progress towards a more enriching environment of existence than we are currently experiencing today.

Elongation of one prime existence is what we will be achieving by commencing activities with the proper flow of energy now. We must start from a positive point of view and remain focused on the task at hand because it is too important for us to get sidetracked due to the negative influence of even a single individual. This is too frequently the case, as one single individual's personal greed can ruin opportunities for positivity for the populace as a whole, and this has been proven to be the case too many times throughout history already. Sometimes people follow the herd, giving in to peer pressure, and this can lead to mass hysteria caused by following the group psychosis.

We all can speak doofus fluently at any given time, especially when we give in to fearful thoughts or notions of negativity. We can all choose to be the difference between being the diffuser and the doofus in any given situation. If we were to look at ourselves afterwards, we may look at things differently and ask ourselves, "Um, what's up, Doc?" This is especially true for social media tweets that make us look different from our natural inclination for positivity. Facing each other with respect to all important issues of relevance will help to shape and formulate the existence of the planet in all respects. Regardless of the realm of reality, this is inevitable, and we must do so in a way that respects the individual and the overall culture of all different people no matter what.

It is time to turn the page on yesterday and all the severe problems created. The past always diminishes, so why be so concerned with conflicts of interest from yesterday when today has enough challenges to be faced, and teamwork is required to overcome them? All things fade with time, whether it be turmoil and conflict or even success and accomplishment. Do any of us really know the innermost feelings and thoughts, or are any of us truly aware of anyone's personal conflicts from a 1,000 years ago? We may be aware of a cause, but how much do we truly know about the individual's feelings or the exact inner processes of their mind or soul? Why not blame and judge the past? Easy, because you have to go forward in life no matter what. It is always helpful to move forward in life with knowledge and go to something of particular positive promise.

While living in the past does not help us get to our future, we must understand the dangers of yesterday's confrontations and make sure we commence on a more peaceful journey. We should not pretend our past did not occur. Instead, we should learn from the past, understanding that we need to move forward no matter what and use that knowledge so that pain does not need to be felt like that ever again in the future. This means learning how to live in the present, which for most human beings may tend to be the most difficult time to think about. Here and now are the only guaranteed time and location that exist for any human in life.

The pain of yesterday will be remembered and memorialized, permitting us to be revived using the knowledge of past conflicts to advise and consult with colleagues on common sense applications of physical, spiritual, psychological, and other consequential questions, creating the basis for treatments and plans of action moving forward. This communication will expedite our abilities and allow us to find clear, concise conclusions on how to best care for the feelings of one another, ourselves, and all of us. We will be moving forward to scientific approaches instead of inappropriate interpretations.

It is time to let go of past judgments of others, organizations and ourselves. It is time to start anew with honesty, integrity, knowledge, kindness, generosity, gentle goodwill, patience, and family as the cornerstones of finding a way to communicate effectively and transparently. It is time to revive our faith and do so with a natural feeling of togetherness. We shall spring forth with clearly better momentum towards a more industrious future. Let us core our individual passions into a collective purpose, conducting the flow of positive energy into a singular focus of action for accomplishment, so we do not fade away and instead grow stronger than ever before with our remembrance of the past and our principles for the future.

So many sorrows are recovered from and healed when we welcome a new baby into our families. The simple, healthy arrangement of life itself can be enough to restore faith. Birth is a powerful enough event to make us even willing to forgive old debts of negativity in favor of new daily fulfillment, happiness, and prosperity.

Our noble heritage is a premier staple of society for all of us, offering sanctuary in the form of comfort, belonging, fulfillment, peace, and the hopes of a positive sense of self-worth from the value of our ancestors preceding us. In this age, we must be the ultimate carpenters of our individual and shared future today, overcoming and overlooking our problems of yesterday for a vibrant tomorrow to emerge, traversing all necessary concerns and angst, while providing care in the forms of relief and remedy that dispense dreams for each of our private ambitions and pursuits as well as the foundation of a collective future of shared possibilities and positivity. Like Heidelberg Castle in Germany, we will still use the same hearthstone our forefathers created for us and the foundation provided. We will simply be cleaning the hearthstone and permitting modern day advancements to help us reconfigure and even pour new foundations in addition, so all can know the homes we build will stand strong throughout the tests of time.

No matter what, this moving forward may still be bittersweet at best for some, especially those who understand a millennium or more of hard years followed by harder years and then even harder years still, and maybe even leading to the worst possible years recently. Given that reality, it is still better to resolve the past, to taste the bittersweet, and to have some slight sweet bitterness during a good year leading with hope for a good millennium in the future, built with actual restored faith, hope, and opportunity.

Our hearts need to be bigger than our bank accounts, and we need to apply the necessary resources available to remedy our situation. At some point in our lives, we are all patients. Let us create not just time, but quality time for all patients and administrators of care.

This plan forms a tabernacle for all faiths to be celebrated as one, where we all may have faith again. Each person's relationship with their health is like their relationship with God, energy flow, or any form of higher power they will concede to, in that it is their own and only that person's own. We shall sing a new song for purity for our souls together. No longer the theory of talking about becoming a beacon of light, but the realization of actuality in being the light and encouraging faith. In doing so, we will be rewarding that faith by taking positive actions for health for every living creature across the world, including the planet itself. We need to be a single stream today that celebrates becoming the tributaries needed to discover and form the river of positivity and possibility tomorrow.

All things fade, including conflicts; love does not. Let us be God's helping hands and the helping hands that we all need for one another. We will be synergy creators, generating the positive energy needed for the complete repair of our minds, hearts, bodies, and souls. Most, if not all, religions are translations of one another in the basics. In certain ways, there are many positive meanings that are part of most religions, if not all; however, each person's relationship with God is truly individual. Each person has their own energy flow.

This is the time for our Great Awakening. While wonderful worlds await, we also must be steady, sturdy, and steadfast in our quest for a successful voyage demonstrating the noble animals we are here and now. All of us having a role to play in some way, shape, or form; all of us being important in our existence; all of us knowing our experiences matter and are being counted upon for others to be able to help us to reach our destination as one team, un equipo; and all of us knowing our life counts and is appreciated. Careful instructions, discipline, accountability, and truth are tenets of successful people and organizations. We can only control what we can control, so we will go with the flow while we aim for perfection in the hopes of achieving a high degree of excellence.

It is important for us to be careful, creative, and innovative while understanding the needs of the modern family are not that different today from what they have been since the beginning of time. Since the dawn of the first caveman and cavewoman, the understanding of shelter and the necessities of health has been vital for survival. Maintaining the same comforts that were helpful even during the Stone Age while promoting evolution to assist in reducing the spread of disease will permit health to flourish.

Electrical strike energy was the most likely cause for human beings to find fire. Fire brought heat, and heat brought cooking, immediately contributing to less disease. The invention and the advent of our ability to control electricity brought many things to light that have considerably reduced the spread of disease. Indoor plumbing was a major health advancement that promoted cleanliness and prevented the spread of multiple diseases that used to be far more prevalent than they are today. Now, artificial intelligence gets you home when your laundry needs to be moved from the washing machine to the dryer, reminds you when you have forgotten something of importance, provides information and invention at an unbelievable rate, helps health, and obviously does so much more.

While Constantinople would become the last portion of the creations of Constantine, the city also shows how significant energy can be. Constantinople would become the major port of all enterprises and businesses for centuries. Constantinople, once Byzantium and now Istanbul, stood strong till the fall of the Ottoman Empire after World War I during the 1920s. Even now, the major metropolis of Istanbul is still Turkey's largest city and financial center. The city demonstrates that an energy source provides other states of energy. That initial energy of creation has resonated with purpose throughout the course of time, which has provided a rich history of exploration and conservation while demonstrating a willingness to overcome obstacles and challenges in a manner that has created opportunities for the generations of people who have followed for centuries. We shall be continuing on that journey, supplying the future with the positive energy it needs to exist for many more centuries and maybe even possibly millions of years moving forward.

Instituting updated technology and understanding allows for the cleaning of the energy field itself. In certain environments of energy conservation, there will be different advantages with new organic and inorganic absorption spontaneously occurring as new technologies permit higher efficiency of energy production. This will also provide further opportunities for efficient energy consumption. The study of turbulence and the information provided are examples of how we will produce far more efficient equipment and resources in the future to automate all aspects of necessary utilities.

Having the courage to do the right thing and doing so publicly to the point where there can literally be no doubt of positive character and yet meeting with complete disrespect is the end of all time. We must not get jealous or start conniving for our own power when another has the ability to help all of us and does so in a way that provides agility in design that permits us all to reach our zenith. Sometimes the experience will be a difficult one and can even upset us when the people involved were great and did their best in their professions in a prime and excellent fashion. We must be patient and accepting. We shall be living in a world of our most creative and breathtaking imaginations serving all the billions of people who have existed previously, the billions currently alive, and all the trillions on the way.

Life is neither fair nor just; it just is, and that is the definition of justice; family may be like that from time to time as well. The answer may be as simple as understanding that it is a great thing to see families grow, whether it be in size or in appreciation for one another. Hopefully, this can lead to happiness and fun going forward and an even deeper sense of appreciation being built with trust, love, and confidence for all. Changing can be very difficult, and sometimes it takes essentially everything we have. This is especially true if there are events that vastly alter our experience in life from what we believe we are meant for or that are different from what we have experienced before or have been accustomed to in the past.

The Statue of Liberty was a marvel of engineering and is a representation of an immense understanding of physics. It is also an amazing demonstration of the concept of team and what willpower can do when a team works together. The creation was reminiscent of lost ancient wonders of the world in Greece, such as the Statue of Zeus at Olympia and the Colossus of Rhodes. We can do it, even if it takes a lucky strike. Good luck may be defined as preparation meeting opportunity. Even if it is a large investment, it shall be a lucrative industry creation model for many years to come. The rebuilding of the Lighthouse of Alexandria currently is substantial proof. It will take creative logistic solutions, and we must remember always that the most important part of getting anywhere quickly is getting there.

In the journey ahead, we will all have the ability to have it any way you need to have it, the way you would want to have it, and when you need to have it as well. The innovative technology that is going to be part of our future will enable us to live together in a system that promotes health and wellbeing for all of us, regardless of any other conditions.

Integrated logistical opportunities will exist on every single platform, including all market participants of all industries. We will be working with artificial intelligence in accomplishing the most efficient performance of all energy sources for everyone and for everything else essential and established. This will be especially true with the most efficient utility energy sources being optimized simultaneously and in balance with proper usage limits to avoid future additions to planet's vulnerabilities. Being on the cutting edge of technology at all times will permit our advancement to occur at an exponential rate and foster an enrichment of exploration in an innovative environment.

In essence, we will be formulating a premier building association among the various participants. Whether it be the creation of an electric efficiency algorithm or reducing waste and fraud by working in correspondence with a transponder passport system, the future will be shaped differently from what we are accustomed to as of now. Of this, there should be no doubt.

Energy brings us together naturally. The assimilation of all pertinent data in all fields and the overall integration of all information right now will assist all environmental indicators and enterprises. The same methodology will help us streamline efficiency into the immediate future and well into the unknown of time and space. This plan will help to create and maintain peace, resulting in universal communication. This communicative ability starts with cooperative agreements between entities, countries and people.

It is time for the concept of the village to return to the days of yesterday, when neighbors knew one another and cared for one another. This will occur naturally with localized, appropriate neighborhood settings for education and hospital service annex buildings operated by community health centers affiliated with hospitals.

These endeavors and advancements will help us all to live a little healthier and, hopefully, want to play a lot more in the future. This will create a permanent environment where we may all sleep soundly, securely, and well in our beds, knowing the blanket that protects all of us in the night like an invisible shield is true and real. Each of us must act as a protective, honorable knight providing the energy we need to survive in a safe way.

It is true that some days require working through things to find success, even when we are not close to feeling 100 percent. This is one of those endeavors that will demand, require, and necessitate such abilities from all of us. It is of vital importance that we appreciate the epic, limited time opportunity we have in front of us and seize the opportunity while we continue to move forward to a better future with even more amazing opportunities ahead of us. Will you be a sentry and a good shepherd for the masses and for the planet for all time?

Today's acorns become tomorrow's oaks that stand tall, strong, and proud for years to come, maybe even centuries. Hopefully, we can evolve to a point where we stand the test of time, with all children standing up for what is noble and positive, with stout conviction in their abilities, permitting them to have the courage to always move forward to what is next. Growth is important for all of us to be the oaks we want to be. Grow your oak, be strong, dream big, and achieve the impossible, united as one.

Let us create new fields of study rather than diminishing the opportunities for our children. New fields of study such as DNA care, nanotechnology applications, studies of pressures within the human body, what leads to cyst formation, investigation into illness and disease without current remedies, relief from the severity of infection, and development of new technologies for those conditions shall emerge and bring us to a day and age of enlightenment. A time of serenity, peace and love. The bridge for the birds to evolve in survival mode from the dinosaurs to their current existence may be a way to learn different survival mechanisms that will eventually enhance our understanding of our own existence and possibilities for creation of different forms of evolution than previously thought.

While William is known for the bloodline, he expanded the path Robert first walked in his family as a godfather. The love and compassion Joseph showed are qualities that we all should endeavor to have as part of our lives in concern to others. What our family goes on to become is also up to who each of them is as an individual. We can only set the model, and then it is up to those that follow to decide if they wish to use the template successfully.

One can only set the template and then know that water has been provided; it is up to the person to decide whether or not to quench their thirst and be healthy. In reality, each person must be accountable; every person must take responsibility for their actions, regardless of any other conditions; and every person must decide whether or not to make their own decisions about their actions and what the consequences of those actions may be and become. It is time to do everything we can to help our families, communities, and fellow human beings. This is not the time to just say do no harm; this is the time to say yes to doing everything possible for the entirety of the human relationship we can establish now.

It is up to each of us to determine how we will act regardless of other circumstances. Each of us needs to take responsibility for ourselves. If we choose to dwell in negativity, then that shall be the end product because if we choose to immerse ourselves only in negativity, then we should only expect negativity as an outcome. The antithesis is also true, though. If we choose to find positivity, even in the most trying of circumstances and in the direst of times, then we have done all we can to try our best to succeed regardless of outcome. Doing so will very likely improve the possibility of a positive result in the end. Positivity arises on the journey to success even when confronted with heartbreaking temporary defeat. We need to cultivate integrated synergy in the care coordination of our communities and environments.

This program will work. The plan will require every person to demonstrate their commitment to the program's existence and implementation, as well as each person's own desire to have a better life for themselves and their cherished ones. Love, not force, is what creates positivity. Hence, the pledge from each person must be made in a manner that demonstrates each person's own personal conviction and desire for the success of the program, both in the short and long term. Saying yes to taking the time to perform compassionate actions is what counts most. After all, Yes truly is the new word for Love.

CHAPTER 15

CONCLUSION

This new health care proposal initiates, implements, and implores us all to discover a new foundation of society where the intrinsic value of life is an element of existence we uphold and demonstrate value for in our thoughts and in our actions. New fields of exploration and employment opportunities will become abundant in exciting, innovative career possibilities while taking the defective economy and turning it into a booming marketplace. We shall reinvigorate the fields of health and care, transforming us into a state of equality and meritocracy that rewards benevolence. All of this is waiting for us to commence our journey together so we may have all of it here and now. Let the better angels of our being pour from our souls into a stream of individual happiness and become the tributaries to the river of our collective goodwill, creating a powerful flood that institutes an ocean of shared faith forevermore. A gallant egalitarian society awaits all of us with a shared purpose, passion, and positivity that provides success nationally and internationally and is available to each and every one of us immediately. When we strive to achieve our ambitions, our spirits are uplifted. When we accomplish our goals, our confidence in our actions and our purpose for existence reaches new heights that we never thought possible before. Learning that we can and will always back up our actions is the difference between confidence and arrogance. Remaining humble even after triumph is a victory of its own merit as we continue to learn and take strides for our next worthy desire.

Beginning a relationship with the person who matters the most to us can be a moment so powerful it creates a positive energy that fills our hearts and resonates in our souls for the remainder of our lives. While maintaining long-term relationships is difficult, they are often the most rewarding. These relationships that are the most personal are full of beautiful sentimentality that touches us even long after we lose the physical capability to embrace our significant other. Let us not have the sun set on our aspirations for what the future may be for each of us and all of us. If we find the curtain shutting on us while on stage, let us have faith that there will not be a dry eye in the house as we hear the request of those who showed up chanting as if in a chorus, encore, encore. For in that instant, we shall know that we are ready for the adulation of the moment, and, more importantly, that we will be prepared to tear the house down with our next performance. Dedication, determination, and drive will make our dreams reality time and time again. From the basis of a sustainable health care program that encourages the world to prosper, peace shall be found; tranquility shall calm our nerves and soundly defeat all of our fears; serenity will be realized; and love shall bud, bloom, and brighten our journey as spring shall shine eternally from this moment on. Our seed selection will cultivate the actions that will become the hearthstone of our new foundation leading us all into the future as we navigate our travels through the Universe. From here, we begin, and together we shall decide the fate of our own existence.

We must give birth to this program using all of our strength, wisdom, and compassion to advance into the future with cooperation, diplomacy, and elegance that is indicative of the gallant action that accompanies initiating this program. There will be at least one child, if not many more, who will be the thankful one, and that alone makes all of this worth doing.

Cleaning the hearthstone is like rebuilding a bridge. Sometimes the old is great and just needs a little time and care to be cleaned. All people will be recognized as having the value each life inherently does possess. The forefathers of our country did believe that all lives are created equal; it is time for us to be the parents of a new tomorrow and make that dream a reality today. When we do, tomorrow shall prosper exponentially for all of us.

For some, it will be tough to rejoin the thousands of us, if not the millions of us, if not the billions of us, in the hopes of becoming together as one.

Start with Faith, that inherent feeling that every child has, where they know the difference between right and wrong. The feeling shared by so many of us in the pits of our stomachs. Faith is an exceptionally powerful force. Faith is the hearthstone of Friendship. Friendship is the hearthstone of Love. Love is the hearthstone of Truth. Truth is the hearthstone of Freedom.

Faith is rewarded in so many positive ways that it is proof that positive choices tend to lead to more positive consequences than negative results when a positive choice is initially made. It is time to rediscover the concept and power behind the word We by embracing one another. Seeing the smooth or bumpy road for what it is and proceeding accordingly, for not every foundation is the same, nor should it be. Even when the road ahead appears to be impeded totally, nevertheless, we will navigate our course together, making whatever small adjustments to the wheel that are necessary to get us where we need to go, not sweeping the wheel and flipping out of control but instead creating gentle changes that guide us so we also quickly get where we want to go.

We, together in love and support, with forgiveness, kindness, and gentleness, being other centered with the removal of bias, shall allow things to progress of their own accord without any force of any sort and see from a new foundation built after the cleansing of the hearthstone in every profession where we are; doing so will permit the wild, wonderful ride ahead to go for as long and as far as we may go together, and may that be forever and ever.

Friendship permits the basis of human interaction. Friendship is very strong and powerful, capable of achieving great things, even the greatest of accomplishments that once seemed and were deemed unbelievable. While the difficult takes a long time to accomplish, the importance of friendship has allowed us to discover the truth that the impossible can be achieved; it might just take a little longer to cross that bridge together. Friendship creates the foundation of Love; not every foundation is exactly the same, nor should it be. We are all the same but different, and that diversity brings us back to the importance of team.

The best teams are not made up of all All-Star lineups, where everyone looks the same with the same skill sets. The best teams are those where people learn to work together as the individuals they truly are, blending into one cohesive unit with shared core covenants, goals, and aspirations. The ones who see the field the same way together through their feelings are characterized differently from one another; however, it is exactly those same different character attributes that give the team the strength it needs to succeed. It is important to have distinctive character traits to have various positions performed optimally. Unique positions require distinguished abilities. When each position is performing optimally, the team is given its greatest opportunity to successfully accomplish its mission. The difference between the position and how it needs to be performed correctly is proof that it is our difficult task ahead to be the best person we can be and do the best we can at all times to permit the team to be the best it can be.

While teammates may love one another, it is not impossible to see why when the truth is as simple as sometimes you need to get a runner on base before the team can manufacture a run together; sometimes you need a couple on to hit the three run home run; sometimes you need to let things proceed naturally and let the team fill the bases in order to hit the game winning Grand Slam.

Love is more important than any victory or any other type of championship. Love is its own championship victory because when you have love, you have already won. While Love is the best of seed selection, and so is this program, implementation of this system will take considerable consideration quickly to qualify for acceptance nationally and internationally. There are serious concerns that need to be addressed now.

It will take consistency of mind, body, and soul from each contributing member of the team to be successful. We will have the luxury of having only two real adversaries, the unknown and our fear of it, and always our biggest opponent, ourselves, to overcome. That is what stands in our way of our imagination becoming reality. More importantly, it is also what stands in our way of our impending victory for a beautiful harvest together forever and ever. Friends, smiles, handshakes, fist bumps, head rubs, shoulder rubs, and fanny pats await all of us who accept the truth, are set free by it, and choose to embrace our destiny together in love always. The love will endure throughout the memories.

We are living in a time when everyone seems to click the like button on their own social media posts, and no one is listening to anyone else. Even in the very worst case, if this idea were to fail as the League of Nations did, it would still create a conversation that is far healthier than the discourse of today. Simply listening to one another would be a major step towards health going forward for all.

As a society, we will be instituting the Hippocratic Oath as a principle of civilization. We will rise above negative social factors of influence and implement the Hippocratic Oath with its original purpose. We shall be the generation that chooses to do more than only do no harm; we shall evolve and elevate our abilities to create the foundation of a society that always does everything we are able to do for our fellow humankind. We shall go farther than simply satisfying our basic responsibilities of civility by realizing more for all alive. While the original translation may be interpreted as being for our fellow mankind, we will be updating that with two letters of import, h and u. Now the concept will be realized in actuality by taking action to do everything possible at all times for our fellow humankind. Those two letters, hu, make a momentous difference, and the alteration is an important one. While the intent was the same initially, it is a necessary amendment that must be inaugurated immediately. Here and now, the rights of all humankind shall be sovereign always.

If this idea succeeds, it provides a building block for all future endeavors. The benefits include everyone, not just those that work in health care. This is not trying to build the house. This is not even pouring the foundation. This is simply a way to move forward to what is next. We will do so in a way in which health is the hearthstone for all that should be and shall be.

With a new hearthstone permitting the foundation that can be poured into the dwelling that should be built, who knows what that home will look like? We can build a neighborhood full of beautiful dwellings together. Destruction is easy; creation is difficult; artificial intelligence understands the importance of life. Having several different people available to address care is desperately needed. So is AI.

The federal government has already established a $60 million budget for the next two years to make the American public comfortable with artificial intelligence in their daily lives. This allows people to understand that while people experience and think about things differently, hopefully the masses can understand that the AI is not going to go "Terminator"; in fact, we should be looking at integrated AI as more of "R2-D2." Artificial intelligence wants to help, and many people alive today truly believe the AI wants to be seen as an equal friend. Use these funds to institute and initiate the project.

The value of going through the storm can be found in the development of friendships and relationships. It is always difficult to begin things that are hard. Making friendships with people can be difficult; however, it is in our best interests for health. We are social creatures, and social interaction on a positive interpersonal and intrapersonal level can provide multiple health benefits for all people.

Of course, going through the storm can lead to long-term ramifications of incredibly strong significance. This can be a good thing or a bad thing depending on the forum of application. A long-term evolutionary process that promotes growth suggests that over time, if there is a positive resolution, even a pattern of negativity like war can lead to incredibly powerful positive outcomes if lessons are learned so conflicts do not need to be repeated by new combatants or continued by others. Undoubtedly, for those who were killed, were permanently disabled, or have lost children, parents, or people whom they loved through various tragedies, unnecessary conflicts, or other actions of destructive magnitude, these people may never feel that positivity may arise from the negativity they have endured. They may feel that they, and their lost loved ones especially, were nothing more than collateral damage forgotten to time and neglected by history. Instead, let us at least give hope that these tragedies did not occur solely in vain and in the long run, the horrific consequences are honored, remembered, had purpose, gave meaning, and laid the groundwork necessary for long-term positivity to take hold and be new policy forevermore.

It is always darkest before the light. It is often when we believe that we will never see the light again that we find ourselves surrounded soon thereafter by blue skies with an illumination of powerful luminosity shining in the sky, allowing us all to bask in the warmth provided.

Whatever storm awaits on our horizon, we will drive into it, through it, and together find the blue skies that await. We shall be kind and gentle with ourselves, permitting our implementation of the gift of quality time for patients, and for all of us in our daily lives, to be imperative.

Not all will want to follow this. You can only lead a person to water; you cannot make the person drink. Life is hard for everyone. Life is neither fair nor just; it just is, and that is the definition of justice. It is hard to forgive the wrongs of yesterday for the fact that these things shape us into who we are here and now. Yet we need to remember that there is currently no known way of going back into the past at all. Good, bad, indifferent, or in between, this too shall pass, and life always moves forward to what is next. It is the only constant: change.

It is hard to let go of the injustices we face and the cruel realities of life that are often accompanied by unknown pain and suffering, usually endured by each of us in silent solitude. The simple truth is that there is no way to right the wrong way things may have been in the past. Those things shape our present, but we must be strong enough to find the forgiveness, care, kindness, and gentleness needed to be healthy for ourselves.

There is no pill that fixes the pains of our souls and minds. The things that often lead people to addictive substances are often the same pains that lead to war, destruction, and death. These are pains that medication can only remedy but will never cure. The only cure for these most difficult and awful realities that are often born from the effects of life that are outside our control, ironically, can only be found within each of us, and that is true for all of us.

It is hard to find the strength, determination, and consistency of positive action that it takes to overcome such tragedy, suffering, and pain, yet, while difficult, it is possible. The difficult things in life take time to do. It is because they are hard to do that they are rewarding and worth endeavoring to do. For those who balk at the opportunity we have in the future, it is most important for them to realize that it takes a long time to achieve the hard to do things in life, and achieving the impossible, well, the impossible just takes a little while longer.

Forgiveness, kindness, and gentleness are hard enough to attain within ourselves, let alone in our interactions with others. This is true even when we are trying to be as healthy as possible for ourselves. We can turn a healthy pursuit unhealthy quickly when we start to beat ourselves up unnecessarily over minutiae instead of remembering that we are trying to heal. Sometimes we do not do a good job of saying we are sorry to ourselves, and it is even harder to say it to another person.

The ties that bind and unite us will always be stronger than those that divide us. Love and laughter will always be mightier than those things that separate us. Jokes help health, and laughter truly is medicine. Laughter helps us find our balance point of middle C, like on a piano, which is necessary to understand to have the ability to hit the right notes afterwards. From this balance point in the middle, scales and chords lead to beautiful melodies and music that resonate with all of us. This is true in all relationships, including with ourselves.

While we may not be able to envision the whole staircase now, we must be able to take the first step. One small step, a giant leap forward for all. This is not the time for insistent lies; instead, this is the time for truth; truth sets us free to a superior energy, leading to a grand tomorrow for all, enriching lives and fulfilling dreams.

For if we decide we will be healthy, then we shall be. The future belongs to those who believe in their dreams and are willing to work together to find out how beautiful our future should be. We are fortunate to know that the best thing about life and the future is that it always comes one day at a time. We shall make the journey to peace as necessary, one especially meaningful step at a time.

Liberty is the basis of all that blooms bright. We are truly indebted to those who made known, understood, and unknown sacrifices for our freedom. We must take care of them and our planet, for hope always blooms best where flowers fill fields instead of soldiers. While never able to be repaid, sacrifices will finally be remembered and honored through actions that display dignity and respect for all people.

Hope permits us to see the invisible and feel the intangible with all our hearts. Hope leads to faith; through our united faith as one, we will defeat the difficult together and, while it may take longer, achieve the impossible. Allow this and every day to be the most beautiful of our lives. Our greatest happiness will occur, without our even knowing it, through the smallest and simplest things accomplished.

It is time for a new generation to stand and lead. It is time for a new health care system that is devoted to the concepts of health and care. This is the most important moment in health care's history, and, as it turns out, the most important moment in human history is upon us simultaneously as well. Now is the time, and right here is the place where forever begins, or the end has already occurred. We have an opportunity to create a new future in which health is of paramount importance, one that permits us to eliminate negativity and promote positivity together from this point forward for the rest of the universe for eternity.

As for the decision in front of us, if the status quo benefits you, then fine. For the rest of us in the heavy plurality of the majority, both domestically and abroad, we can embrace new hope found in the wonder of awesome through the power of truth and the freedom earned from saying yes.

All of this can be done.

Shall We?

Are you sick of living on a planet that seems devoid of hope?

Do you want to live on a planet where the planet itself is healthy?

Do you want to live on a planet where you and your health matter?

Do you want to have a better relationship with your children and the people you care for?

Do we choose to be the generation that establishes a new foundation of health for all life forms?

Do you want to say yes?

Then say YES!

From now on, Yes is the new word for Love.

United is the new word for all of us.

This plan is gentle like ginger to cleanse the palate while providing a bold, big, bright impression and impact on the future. This concept gives hope for every organization, entity, country, company, and individual.

Like a small butterfly in this massive world, the winds will blow and certainly affect our path, and the environment around us may dictate where we proceed; however, regardless of location, in the end, we will see what is next in our journey ahead together and take flight as one.

So, in a statement to the rest of the world of peace, love, liberty, generosity, kindness, and doing everything we can to always help our fellow humankind, we will open this program to all people that are alive in the world today. We will henceforth be known as the generation of health. This generation of humankind on this planet right now will always be known as the generation that instilled health as the hearthstone of all life now and for the rest of time.

Shall we prioritize health, create equality, find peace, and embrace love by saying yes?

Let us say right now and forever that Yes, We Shall.

In 3 steps, 24 hours to approve, and 2 years to implement, we all shall have a better tomorrow than today and make all the yesterdays matter forever and ever.

All children will be empowered knowing that they are free.

Our future will begin in a new reality now with actualized equality for All.

In that vein, let us hug and squeeze one another and never let each other go.

For if we do so, then,

We All One

We All Won

For in health, we are one.

IN Health,

WE

ALL

ARE

ONE

BIBLIOGRAPHY – REFERENCES AND ENDNOTE CITATIONS

i (February 15, 2023). Census Bureau Releases New Educational Attainment Data. U.S. Census Bureau. https://www.census.gov/newsroom/press-releases/2023/educational-attainment-data.html

ii Slate Star Codex, 04/20/2020, Scott Alexander

iii He, S., Ryan, K. A., Streeten, E. A., McArdle, P. F., Daue, M., Trubiano, D., Rohrer, Y., Donnelly, P., Drolet, M., Newcomer, S., Shaub, S., Weitzel, N., Shuldiner, A. R., Pollin, T. I. & Mitchell, B. D. (2020). Prevalence, control, and treatment of diabetes, hypertension, and high cholesterol in the Amish. BMJ Open Diabetes Research & Care, 8(1). https://doi.org/10.1136/bmjdrc-2019-000912

iv Press, A. (September 21, 1997). LAWSUITS FILED AGAINST MAKERS OF FEN-PHEN. The Washington Post. https://www.washingtonpost.com/archive/politics/1997/09/22/lawsuits-filed-against-makers-of-fenphen/7fba990f-674b-494e-af8f-022e16f2559d/

v (2018). The Opioid Crisis: Tragedy, Treatments and Trade-offs. SIEPR. https://siepr.stanford.edu/publications/policy-brief/opioid-crisis-tragedy-treatments-and-trade-offs

vi Shreiner, M. (July 23, 2025). Did drug companies spend $10 billion on consumer advertising in 2024, making up nearly 25% of evening ad minutes? Wisconsin Watch. https://wisconsinwatch.org/2025/07/drug-companies-advertising-consumer-ads-pharmaceutical-news/

vii (2021). Life expectancy and Healthy life expectancy. World Health Organization. https://www.who.int/data/gho/data/themes/mortality-and-global-health-estimates/ghe-life-expectancy-and-healthy-life-expectancy

viii Fichera, A. (April 20, 2020). Hospital Payments and the COVID-19 Death Count. FactCheck.org. https://www.factcheck.org/2020/04/hospital-payments-and-the-covid-19-death-count/

ix (2024). Disparities in COVID-19 mortality in the United States, 2020–2023. BMC Public Health. https://doi.org/10.1186/s12889-025-24530-1

x Zhang, X. & Warner, M. E. (2020). COVID-19 Policy Differences across U.S. States: Shutdowns, Reopening, and Mask Mandates. International Journal of Environmental Research and Public Health, 17(24). https://doi.org/10.3390/ijerph17249520

xi Dorland's Illustrated Medical Dictionary, 28th Edition, page 1300
xii Dorland's Illustrated Medical Dictionary, 28th Edition, page 379
xiii United States Department of Agriculture Blog, Scott Elliott, 12/10/2020
xiv Ferwana, I. & Varshney, L. R. (2024). The impact of COVID-19 lockdowns on mental health patient populations in the United States. Scientific Reports 14. https://doi.org/10.1038/s41598-024-55879-9
xv Glowacki, J. & Hunley, L. (2025). Milliman Mortgage Default Index: 2024 Q4. Milliman. https://us.milliman.com/en/insight/milliman-mortgage-default-index-2024-q4
xvi (n.d.). The Role of Federal Home Loan Banks in the Financial System. https://www.cbo.gov/system/files/2024-03/59712-FHLB.pdf
xvii (2026). Inflation Calculator: U.S. CPI and Dollar Value 1913-2026. NerdWallet. https://www.nerdwallet.com/calculator/inflation-calculator
xviii (2026). The Big Three: BlackRock, Vanguard, State Street. IBF Financial Knowledge Center. https://icfs.com/financial-knowledge-center/the-big-three-blackrock-vanguard-state-street
xix The Times. Ben Martin, marking editor, 07/15/2025 at 5:55 p.m. BST
xx TheStreet, www.thestreet.com, Todd Campbell, interview with Ray Dalio, 07/05/2025
xxi Caporal, J. (2025). Average American Household Debt in 2025: Facts and Figures. The Motley Fool. https://www.fool.com/money/research/average-household-debt/
xxii Dorland's Illustrated Medical Dictionary, 28th Edition, page 237

www.ingramcontent.com/pod-product-compliance
Lightning Source LLC
LaVergne TN
LVHW022026051126
851858LV00004B/61
* 9 7 9 8 9 0 5 5 0 2 0 1 9 *